O9-CFS-980

Praise for *The Real Food Revolution*

"Congressman Tim Ryan isn't afraid to take on a challenge, and he's gearing up for one of America's biggest—our health. In *The Real Food Revolution*, he delivers a straightforward and much-needed prescription to help transform our country's food systems and improve our well-being."

—President Bill Clinton

"In *The Real Food Revolution*, Congressman Tim Ryan not only puts a spotlight on everything wrong with our current food system, he also lays out a bold but realistic plan to give every American access to fresh, whole foods, and gives specific steps we all can take to join the food revolution that is happening now across America."

—Arianna Huffington, editor-in-chief of the Huffington Post and author of *Thrive*

"It's wonderful that Congressman Tim Ryan cares about the way food affects the health of Americans. I just wish more members of Congress cared about these issues, too."

—Marion Nestle, professor of nutrition, food studies, and public health at New York University and author of *Food Politics*

"As someone who's been on the frontlines of medicine, I've seen the health of our population take a negative turn—and one of the key reasons for this is our less-than-optimal food supply. That's why *The Real Food Revolution* is so important. It gives you the background to understand what's wrong and concrete things you can do to fix the problem. It's time to take back our health and Congressman Ryan is leading the way."

—Andrew Weil, M.D., *New York Times* best-selling author of *True Food* and *Spontaneous Happiness*

"Congressman Tim Ryan reminds us of the old Irish saying, 'Is this a private fight, or can anyone get in?' He wants all of America—through our shopping, gardening, advocacy, and voting—to force a better farm bill, a more responsible food industry, and better diets and health for all of us."

—United States Senator Sherrod Brown, member of the Senate Committee on Agriculture, Nutrition, and Forestry

"*The Real Food Revolution* addresses the most significant problem we face today. We are what we eat, and what we eat is being tampered with in a gigantic way. Our very survival is at stake, but we finally have a courageous voice in the halls of congress who is willing to say 'enough is enough' and offer constructive ways to avert a potential disaster if we fail to act now. I wholeheartedly encourage everyone to read this book and take action."

—Dr. Wayne W. Dyer, *New York Times* best-selling author of *I Can See Clearly Now* and *The Power of Intention*

"*The Real Food Revolution* is a big breath of fresh air and common sense. Its message is urgent and accurate. And written in plain English by a very courageous congressman. Read it."

—Christiane Northrup, M.D., ob/gyn, physician, and author of the *New York Times* bestsellers *Women's Bodies, Women's Wisdom* and *The Wisdom of Menopause*

"Congressman Tim Ryan shows us how to break free from a failing food system. Hopefully this call for action will finally wake up the government agencies that are asleep at the wheel."

—Vani Hari, FoodBabe.com

"In his book *The Real Food Revolution,* Tim shares a simple but profound message that we have the power to improve the quality of our health and life, both individually and collectively. By becoming a little more conscious and knowledgeable about our choices as consumers and devoting a little time and organizing effort, we can truly effect a food revolution that will transform our national diet and the food supply chain supporting it. I believe this book has credibility not only because Representative Tim Ryan can relate to the typical American food cravings, but more importantly because he understands the inertia of the government and industrial interests and the levers of change involved to effectively create the food revolution we so desperately need."

—Deepak Chopra, M.D., *New York Times* best-selling author of *The Future of God*

"Congressman Tim Ryan inspires us with his passion for healthy food, grown, prepared, and cooked with love. He skewers legislation that favors the fat-cat food industry and damages our health. And, he offers a transformative and deeply satisfying vision for a healthy, economically sound national food policy. *The Real Food Revolution* is the real deal."

—James S. Gordon, M.D., founder and director of The Center for Mind-Body Medicine and author of *Unstuck: Your Guide to the Seven-Stage Journey Out of Depression*

"Tim Ryan recognizes the complex web we live in, where agriculture, nutrition, environment, and community intersect and intertwine. In his conversational, insightful, and far-ranging *The Real Food Revolution*, he not only lays out the problems we face but offers simple, commonsense solutions for readers to take action in their own lives and promote positive change on a grander scale."

—Frank Lipman, M.D., founder of the Eleven Eleven Wellness Center and author of *Revive*

"Tim Ryan admits that we're all in the same boat when it comes to being unhealthy in America. We have the deck stacked against our well-being with unhealthy food choices coming from all sorts of out-of-balance practices that bring food to our plates. *The Real Food Revolution* empowers us as individuals to save our nation in crisis, one meal at a time."

—Tara Stiles, founder of Strala Yoga and author of *Make Your Own Rules Diet*

"Food is a complex, emotional, and nostalgic subject that weaves its way through so many aspects of our lives. And it's never been more important to vote with our dollars to influence not only our own personal health but also our national policies and consciousness around healthier, more sustainable food choices. Enter *The Real Food Revolution*. Congressman Tim Ryan paints an entertaining and elucidating portrait of our national obsession with cheap, unhealthy food and provides passionate, actionable solutions for change. This book is a powerful call to action for Americans to collectively create a better future for our country by starting with what's on our plates."

—Jason Wrobel, host of *How to Live to 100* on Cooking Channel and celebrity vegan chef

"I highly recommend *The Real Food Revolution* to everyone who cares about their health and our world's food supply. Congressman Tim Ryan brings us hope and realistic solutions. I'm deeply grateful and impressed by Tim Ryan's courage to speak the truth about politics and food corporations. He is a true leader among politicians and people."

—Doreen Virtue, best-selling author of
The Art of Raw Living Food

"We're eating ourselves to death. Finally a legislator with real solutions rather than hollow platitudes."

—James and Claudia Altucher, authors of
The Power of No

"It is refreshing to find a politician taking a definitive stance on food issues in America. Congressman Ryan is a true role model for America's present and future citizens and leaders. I look forward to a real food revolution finding its way into homes, classrooms, and communities across the United States—and influencing American agriculture from our policies to our plates!"

—Meredith Hill, English language arts educator and garden coordinator at Columbia Secondary School
for Math, Science, and Engineering

THE
REAL
FOOD
REVOLUTION

Also by Tim Ryan

A Mindful Nation:
How a Simple Practice Can Help Us Reduce Stress, Improve
Performance, and Recapture the American Spirit

Please visit:

Hay House USA: www.hayhouse.com®
Hay House Australia: www.hayhouse.com.au
Hay House UK: www.hayhouse.co.uk
Hay House South Africa: www.hayhouse.co.za
Hay House India: www.hayhouse.co.in

THE REAL FOOD REVOLUTION

HEALTHY EATING, GREEN GROCERIES, and the Return of THE AMERICAN FAMILY FARM

Congressman
TIM RYAN

HAY HOUSE, INC.
Carlsbad, California • New York City
London • Sydney • Johannesburg
Vancouver • Hong Kong • New Delhi

Copyright © 2014 by Tim Ryan

Published and distributed in the United States by: Hay House, Inc.:
www.hayhouse.com® • *Published and distributed in Australia by:*
Hay House Australia Pty. Ltd.: www.hayhouse.com.au • *Published
and distributed in the United Kingdom by:* Hay House UK, Ltd.:
www.hayhouse.co.uk • *Published and distributed in the Republic of
South Africa by:* Hay House SA (Pty), Ltd.: www.hayhouse.co.za • *Distributed in Canada by:* Raincoast Books: www.raincoast.com • *Published in India by:* Hay House Publishers India: www.hayhouse.co.in

Cover design: Karla Baker • *Interior design:* Riann Bender

All rights reserved. No part of this book may be reproduced by
any mechanical, photographic, or electronic process, or in the form of
a phonographic recording; nor may it be stored in a retrieval system,
transmitted, or otherwise be copied for public or private use—other
than for "fair use" as brief quotations embodied in articles and re-
views—without prior written permission of the publisher.

The author of this book does not dispense medical advice or prescribe the use of any technique as a form of treatment for physical,
emotional, or medical problems without the advice of a physician,
either directly or indirectly. The intent of the author is only to offer
information of a general nature to help you in your quest for emotional and spiritual well-being. In the event you use any of the information in this book for yourself, the author and the publisher assume
no responsibility for your actions.

Cataloging-in-Publication Data is on file at the Library of Congress

Hardcover ISBN: 978-1-4019-4638-8

10 9 8 7 6 5 4 3 2 1
1st edition, October 2014

Printed in the United States of America

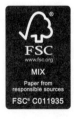
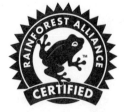

To Mason, Bella, and Brady, and all our children, on whose health the prosperity of our nation depends.

CONTENTS

FOREWORD

I've never read a call to action like this that was written by a politician. People like you and me are usually the ones who are trying to get politicians to listen to us—not the other way around. Well, Tim Ryan is different. He's not only a refreshing new voice in the food revolution but also a bright star who can lead us to the kind of healthy future we dream of for ourselves and our children.

But here's the thing. Tim needs us. He needs us to stay open minded as we read this factual and well-researched book (made easier to digest by his humor and heart). He also needs us to take action. Baby steps. Giant leaps. Whatever we've got the time and fire for. I don't know about you, dear reader, but I want to be on the courageous side of history. Not the right or wrong side, not the Democratic or Republican side, but the side that sees the problems and has the fortitude to organize and deliver thoughtful solutions.

You may think the issues Tim talks about in these pages will only affect future generations or are of no concern to you for some other reason—I certainly thought that way once. However, the future is now and the interconnected politics of our food system and health care impact each and every one of us.

My wake-up call to these issues and to wellness took place when I got really sick. Isn't that how many transformative shifts take place? We're just going about the business of living when a serious diagnosis, a divorce, the loss of a loved one, or financial trouble stops us in our tracks. These turning points force us to make changes. Ultimately many of those changes can have a positive impact, especially if we're willing to adopt a resilient mentality and dig in to the task at hand.

For me, the task was learning to live with an incurable yet slow-growing cancer. I was 31 years old when I was diagnosed and I was totally devastated. How could this have happened to me? Cancer didn't even run in my family, and I was reasonably healthy, or so I thought. Tough decisions followed. Would I do extreme treatments that may not improve my situation? Or would I watch and wait and let cancer make the first move, track the disease and try to make a game plan in the process? Some doctors gave me an expiration date. Others thought I could potentially be around for many years. Ultimately I chose to watch and live and do my best to learn how to take care of myself.

And the adventure began . . .

Not long after my diagnosis I became a student of holistic living. I took the "you are what you eat" wisdom to heart and headed straight to the health food store. My eyes were stinging with tears, both from the shock of my diagnosis and the sight of kale. I often joke that I didn't know which was tougher—the cancer or that plant! But over time I taught myself how to cook delicious, wholesome food and upgraded my diet and lifestyle, and I slowly started to feel better and even thrive—with cancer.

Luckily, you don't have to wait until you're up against the ropes to care for yourself. You can start now. Your grocery list is a political manifesto. It's a declaration of health and independence, and it's worth fighting for. Take it from me; prevention is the best cure. And it happens on our plates, through our lifestyle practices, and whether or not we love and value our selves, our communities, and the world around us.

Change comes from two directions. The bottom up—when folks like you and I join forces, vote with our dollars (and forks), and demand change—and the top down—when forward-thinking politicians like Tim Ryan work across the aisle on our behalf. I couldn't be more proud of this book and more honored to be a part of it. Tim's positivity and passion are like a breath of fresh air. He skillfully lays out the problems and focuses the entire second half of the book on practical, doable solutions.

The Real Food Revolution will help you rise up to the challenge of living a healthier life, and the more of us that do this, the easier it will be to create larger change. We have the power to spread the word about what truly promotes health. We have the power to influence politicians, producers, and distributors to make better food more affordable and accessible. We have the power to step forward on the path of health and bring our loved ones along with us. This book will give you ideas on how to embrace your power. Thank you, Tim Ryan. Thank you for leading the way and being on the courageous side of history.

Kris Carr

PREFACE

*Treat the whole problem of health
in soil, plant, animal, and man as
one great subject.*

—Sir Albert Howard

There is one place where nearly everything that matters today in the world converges: our fork. Food—the way we produce and consume it—is the nexus of most of our world's health, environmental, economic, and even political crises.

Luckily, there are voices out there working to create a food system that bolsters, rather than undermines, our world. They're fighting for what Congressman Tim Ryan calls a *real food revolution*, and that's exactly what Tim so eloquently, simply, and self-evidently describes in this book.

Why would a doctor be so interested in food and food policy?

Here's why.

Never before have we seen a global crisis of chronic disease on the scale we currently face. Lifestyle-caused disease now kills 50 million people a year, more than twice as many as infectious disease. Today, half as many people go to bed hungry as go to bed overweight. And one in two Americans and one in four teenagers has pre-diabetes or type-2 diabetes. We are raising the first generation of Americans who will live sicker and die younger than their parents.

Looking beyond simply our lower quality of life, we can see that our poor health affects our country and our world in larger ways. According to the World Economic Forum, chronic disease is now is the single biggest threat to global economic development. It will cost the world's economy $47 trillion ($47,000,000,000,000) over the next 20 years, more than the annual gross domestic product (GDP) of the six biggest economies combined.

Our children's future is threatened by an achievement gap caused in large part by their inability to learn well after consuming the processed foods and sugar served in schools. Fifty percent of schools serve brand name fast foods in the cafeteria, and 80 percent have contracts with soda companies. Most schools now have only deep fryers and microwaves, which are only able to serve up industrial foodlike substances prepared by corporations, not by humans.

We are also depleting nature's capital—capital that, once destroyed, cannot be reclaimed. One acre of arable land is lost to development every minute of every day. One pound of meat requires 2,000 gallons of water and produces 58 times more greenhouse gasses than 1 pound of potatoes. Our industrial animal factory farms produce more methane and greenhouse gases and use more fossil fuels than all forms of transportation combined (air, car, ship, train). We are destroying our rivers, lakes, and oceans by the runoff of nitrogen-based fertilizers and pesticides. And three quarters of our fresh water is used for agriculture, mostly to grow meat for human consumption. Wars of the future will be fought over water, not oil.

Lobbyists' influence over policy makers has put corporations, not citizens, at the center of every aspect of our food system, from what and how food is grown, to what is manufactured, marketed, and sold. Through our national food policy that subsidizes, protects, and encourages the growth of centralized seed production, mono-crops, and industrial practices, we are systematically destroying both our human and natural capital.

Our most powerful tool to reverse the global epidemic of chronic disease, heal the environment, reform politics, and revive economies is the fork. What we put on it has tremendous implications. Remember, what we do to our bodies, we do to the planet, and what we do to the planet, we do to our bodies.

As a doctor on the front lines of the chronic disease epidemic, it is increasingly clear that food—real, good, healthy food—is the answer. We have come to a tipping point. Industrial, highly processed, hyperpalatable, and highly addictive food is no longer okay. We know better now.

In *The Real Food Revolution,* Congressman Tim Ryan advocates for important policy changes, such as the decentralization of seed production, transparency in food labeling (including GMOs), reduction of antibiotic and hormone use, and rebalancing farm subsidies to give more support to the small and medium specialty farmers who bring real food straight to our tables.

But the real revolution described is this book is local, as local as your fork and what you choose to put on it every single day. As a doctor, it is increasingly clear to me that the health of our nation depends on disruptive innovations that decentralize and democratize food production and consumption. I cannot cure diabetes in my office. It is cured on the farm, in the grocery store, in the restaurant, and in our kitchens, schools, workplaces, and faith-based communities.

Food is the most powerful medicine. Let's teach ourselves and our children about the care and feeding of the human body so we can avert the tsunami of disease and the environmental, social, and economic impact caused by our current food system.

Innovations, pockets of creativity, and decentralized solutions are already happening. We simply need to water the seeds of change. We have to take back our health one kitchen, one home, one family, one community at a time!

Mark Hyman, M.D.

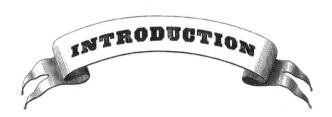

INTRODUCTION

WELCOME TO THE REVOLUTION

Hello. My name is Tim Ryan. I am addicted to chicken wings and ice cream. Ask anyone. My wife, my friends, my acquaintances. Oh yeah. We could finish a huge meal and a half hour later I'll crave a handful of buffalo chicken wings just to wrap up the night.

One night out on the road with my brother Al and some friends, I had an incident. Al was already asleep in the hotel room we were sharing, having gone up to bed not long after dinner. I came in, and, you guessed it, I ordered some chicken wings and a side of ice cream from room service. While I waited for my food I turned on the TV, took off my shirt, and stretched out on the bed. As I flipped through the channels I found the old, original *Batman* TV show. You know, the one with Adam West where Batman and Robin almost die at the end of every episode. Eventually the chicken wings and ice cream arrived. I immediately started eating the wings, piling the bones on a plate next to me on the bed.

Then as I began to put a scoop of ice cream in my mouth something terrible happened. Al rolled over and looked at me with wing sauce on my face and ice cream heading to my mouth. *Busted,* I thought. He then looked at the TV and didn't see an old movie or *SportsCenter*, but a *Batman* rerun from the '60s. He turned back to me with a look only an older brother could give a little brother and said, "What in the hell are you doing?"

Trying to at least sidestep the food issue, I said, "I think this is the final episode. The Joker really has Batman and Robin in the crosshairs."

All he said was, "You got issues," and rolled over and went back to sleep.

I share this story because I want you to know that I am not a purist. I am not an absolutist or an extremist. I love food, and lots of different kinds of food. I go on different diets and then I cheat. Every week I try to watch what I eat—to be good, so that at some point I can be bad. But I have, slowly and over time, moved myself in the direction of healthier eating. I have started to pay more attention, especially now that I am married with a ten-year-old daughter, an eleven-year-old son, and a newborn baby boy.

It seems that everything is so complicated these days, particularly in Washington, DC, which is why I revel in finding something simple to follow. The kind of advice grandmothers give to small children. Like the first words of Michael Pollan's *In Defense of Food: An Eater's Manifesto*: "Eat food. Not too much. Mostly plants." By food, he means whole food, real food, not "food-like substances." I try to do that these days.

While I have had *personal* setbacks like the one with my brother, as a member of the United States Congress I have also watched many *public* setbacks as our government continues policies and strategies that make eating bad food or fake food the most convenient option. I'm guessing you know what I mean by fake food. In fact, I saw some just a few minutes ago at the checkout counter when I was buying some sticky notes and printer paper at Staples. (Yes, we buy food at office supply stores these days. Go figure.) It was a package of super-stuffed "cheese" cracker sandwiches, but there was nothing in it that resembled what my grandparents would have called cheese, and the top ingredients were corn sweetener and oil from soy and some highly processed flour, and then the usual bunch of unpronounceable ingredients to make the snack look more appealing and last until my ten-year-old daughter graduates from college. In America, we love our food. We must, because supplying us with food is very big business. The Fortune 500 companies behind our tasty snacks, prepared meals, and groceries earned $745 billion in 2013, and by 2015 it's estimated that sales for snack foods alone will top $333 billon. We love our food, yes, but I'm not so sure all this food is loving us back.

Why does our food system matter so much to a U.S. Congressman? It matters because cheap, convenient food is costing us a lot in health care costs down the road, and because the most basic resource we require to be a dynamic, innovative country—a nutritious, healthy, reliable food supply—is broken:

- 35 percent of adults are obese
- Obesity has more than doubled in children and quadrupled in adolescents in the past 30 years
- In 2012, more than one-third of children and adolescents were overweight or obese
- In 2012, 15 percent of American households were food insecure, accounting for 49 million Americans—33.1 million adults and 15.9 million children

Simply put, whether it's obesity, food insecurity, or other negative health outcomes from poor nutrition, the majority of Americans are ill-served by our food system. That's a crisis, I'd say.

The kind of food we get and how we get it matters. We have come to the point where the government is effectively "prescribing" a diet for Americans—and prescribing medicine—because the diet is making enough people unwell that they require expensive medication to compensate.

Your tax dollars are making fake food cheaper. Yes, I said it. And it is true. Hardworking families try to make ends meet and also meet their societal obligations by paying taxes. And what does the United States Congress do with that money? It makes fake food artificially cheaper than it would otherwise be in a free market. The massive payments we make to "support" our food system go largely to big producers for corn, soy, and wheat; little goes to smaller, regional farmers producing diversified specialty crops—including fruits and vegetables—in more sustainable and humane ways. And then we eat that food, get sick, and need care, which is often funded by the government through Medicare and Medicaid and the credit available for middle-income families taking part in the Affordable Care Act. So we pay to make cheap food, and then we pay to heal people who eat that cheap food.

About now, you might be thinking, *Uh-oh, this book is just going to bum me out and make me reach for a bag of potato chips, a Coke float, and the TV remote to chill out.* Yes, I do feel the need to share some of the bad news that doctors, farmers, cooks, and advocates for healthier food and a clean environment have shared with me, but I hope this acts not to bum you out, but instead to fire you up. In fact, I think you'll find what I have to say in this book interesting, if not a little shocking. I hope you see it as a wake-up call to help us focus on what we need to do. That's what the first part of this book is about.

But have no fear—things are changing. Part II of this book outlines what I call the real food revolution. Yes, change is already under way. There are amazing people out there doing amazing things. And they started just like you and I. They saw a problem and tried to fix it. And we can all join with them—or step out on our own—to help move our national diet and the supply chain that supports it in the direction of greater health, well-being, and sustainability.

One group of Americans I have great faith in is our family farmers. While I have some criticisms of our overall food system, I have tremendous confidence that our farmers will always supply us with what we desire as consumers. It is our job, as consumers and citizens concerned with the alarming rates of sickness in America, to make sure there is ample demand for specialty crops and other local agricultural products. When consumers demand something, the market will shift. When we demanded safer cars, although it took time, they started to be supplied. When we wanted more fuel-efficient vehicles, people started voting with their dollars and that market began to grow. So we need to make sure we are asking our farmers to grow the kind of food we want for our families and put policies in place that will help grow this market for them to sell to. I am not here to write a pie-in-the-sky book that may sound good yet overlooks the reality of our situation and will never actually move us forward. Who has time for that?

I hope that after reading this book you will join the broader movement of Americans who want to create a big shift in what is sold in our grocery stores and restaurants and at what price.

||||||||||||||||||||||||||||||||||||||||||||||||||||||||||||||||||||||||||||||||||||||||||||||||||||||||||||

The Real Food Revolution is a political book, a community organizing book, a call to action. At the end of each chapter in Part II, I lay out specific things you can do to join the movement—much of it from the comfort of your own home, using the Internet, your phone, or the mail if you like. But if we are going to really make a dent, it is going to take each of us dedicating a little bit of our time to not just visualize what we want the future to look like, but also to organize that future. There are opportunities everywhere. You can even get out and join up with like-minded folks and get your hands dirty (sometimes literally). Let's do this thing!

||||||||||||||||||||||||||||||||||||||||||||||||||||||||||||||||||||||||||||||||||||||||||||||||||||||||||||

Thomas Jefferson is one of my heroes, a guiding light. He envisioned a country ruled by yeoman farmers. He also felt that industrialization, urbanization, and financial speculation would hurt the average citizen. And in a sense, with regard to our food system, he's been proven right. Mass urbanization, for the first time in history, separated large numbers of us from the growing of our food. Industrialization, with all of its benefits, has had some serious consequences as it has been applied to food. While we are never going to be a country where every family owns a few acres to farm and livestock to raise, we can certainly be inspired by Jefferson's vision. He recognized that there was something important in having each citizen somehow tied to the land. He realized that there was something fundamental and virtuous about the process of feeding yourself and putting in the hard work necessary to make it happen.

He wrote, "Cultivators of the earth are the most valuable citizens. They are the most vigorous, the most independent, the most virtuous, and they are tied to their country and wedded to its liberty and interests by the most lasting bonds." There is something spiritual about participating in the process of growing your own food. Anyone who has ever had a garden and spent any time tending to it has felt the connection to the land. It is special.

I'm a Democrat, but that does not limit who I will work with to get the best outcome for America. I'm driven by results and realities, not fixed ideologies. In time-honored Ohio tradition, I am pragmatic. I live by varied perspectives and points of view. In this book, I am not advocating for the abolishment of the agriculture industry as it stands today. I'm not calling for extensive new regulations. Just a few key changes. Like Michael Moss, *New York Times* best-selling author of *Salt Sugar Fat,* I don't view the food industrial complex as "an evil empire that intentionally set out to make us overweight or ill." Individually, they probably mean no harm, but their practices are doing great harm nonetheless. That's undeniable.

CALLS TO ACTION

We need nutrition, agricultural, and environmental reform in this country. And all reform begins with a call to action. Martin Luther King, Jr., brought the issue of racial injustice into every living room in America with his "I have a dream" speech. The first phase of the environmental movement was spurred by Rachel Carson's exposé of DDT in *Silent Spring.* Ralph Nader changed the face of the auto industry with *Unsafe at Any Speed. An Inconvenient Truth* moved a generation of people to care about climate change. These movements are far from over, but we are better off because of them. And now, we have the beginnings of a real food revolution. Many of the people I will mention in this book are pioneers in this movement.

- Morgan Spurlock's 2004 documentary *Super Size Me* called attention to the issue of the ill effects of fast food in a graphic (and sometimes funny) way

- In 2008, Robert Kenner's documentary *Food, Inc.,* symbolized by a cow in a pasture with a UPC code covering the side of its body, gave us a close look at the extent of corporate control of our food system

- In 2009, *Fresh* helped to further propel a grassroots effort to make changes toward a healthier food system, and introduced us to many of the movement's early leaders

- *National Geographic* started a major undertaking with their May 2014 issue: to spend the next eight issues focusing on "The Future of Food," with a deeply researched collection of articles, photographs, and videos

- The documentary *Fed Up,* released in May from Katie Couric and Laurie David, is providing a potent manifesto for the real food revolution

I also understand that the world faces the daunting challenge of doubling our food production by 2050. In order to feed nine billion people, we will need innovative food science; locavore solutions will not meet every need. But relying on a system that is making us sick and damaging our environment is no solution at all.

I believe in self-care and taking personal responsibility. That's a key American value. I do not blame the citizen—the average consumer or taxpayer—for not being able to navigate a system that is rigged against them. The American agricultural and nutritional crisis will not be solved by scolding people for their lifestyle—a lifestyle that is celebrated by massive marketing campaigns and underwritten by Uncle Sam.

My friends across the aisle in the Republican party like to quote my hero Jefferson back to me, as they advocate "getting the government off of everyone's back." But what I'm advocating is completely in line with Jeffersonian values. I, along with others in this movement, want to empower the average citizen to make choices for the good of themselves and for the good of us all. I want to allow more people to be independent producers, not so beholden to big monopolies. That's the oldest kind of American value.

We need to move toward the future by grounding ourselves in our founding values. There is not a more important, agreed-upon value than the one that says that good food should be safe, nourishing, affordable, accessible, and unharmful to the environment. After 12 years in the United States Congress, it's my belief that there is nothing on the political agenda that can unite us as a country, across the current Democrat/Republican divide, like the acknowledgment of the failures of our current system and the damage it's doing to the health and well-being of our nation.

There are few issues that can bring us together more than a new approach to how we subsidize, grow, distribute, and prepare our food. The raging popularity of food shows, blogs, and speakers and the growth of the healthy eating movement demonstrate just how interested we are in food, and how much we care. In cities all over America, citizens are coming together to transform their communities.

Let's water these seeds that have been planted by the pioneers in the real food revolution, and work together to grow a system that promotes fresh local food; encourages small, regional family farms that are good for the environment; and puts local folks to work close to home. As we tear down old dilapidated neighborhoods across America, let's promote farms and gardens in our urban and suburban areas. Let's teach our kids how to grow, cook, and prepare healthy food. Who knows? Perhaps we can inspire them to pursue a career in sustainable agriculture and help us scale up this revolution.

We need every citizen who wants better, cheaper food for themselves and their children to help support policies that can make this happen. We need to think of whole foods as more than the name of a major food chain. It should be something available to all, at affordable prices. Each of us needs to pay a little more attention so that our tax dollars don't go to foolish programs that literally make us sick. The hardworking moms of America are a powerful bunch. They are Democrats, Republicans, and Independents. And they recognize the dangerous trends and the huge problems we'll be leaving our children if we do not act fast. Let's come together with the tens of millions of other like-minded Americans who want to promote health and wellness in different areas of society and reshape the American landscape—and the food that's growing there.

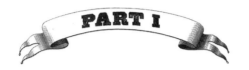

PART I

THE
PROBLEM

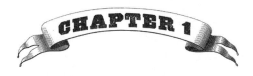

OUR FAILING HEALTH

Our food is making us sick and we need to change that. Or our children's quality of life will be severely diminished.

> *Our food dollars can either go to support a food industry devoted to quantity and convenience and "value" or they can nourish a food chain organized around values— values like quality and health.*
>
> —Michael Pollan

The other day, on my way to a place in the country where I was spending a few days working on this book, on a two-mile stretch of road on the outskirts of a small town, I counted 14 fast food outlets, with full parking lots. I picked up a local paper. There were flyers from four different food stores advertising their weekly specials. I counted:

- 47 sales on soda and sugary drinks
- 41 sales on pastries, cookies, and candy
- 47 sales on snack foods and sugary cereals

There were many two-for-one deals. There were also sales on meat, vegetables, and fruit, but the packaged processed foods dominated the pages. I haven't become a food snob; I've eaten plenty of these things in my time, and, every once in a great while during moments of weakness, I still do. But as I look at the food environment my children are growing up in, I'm increasingly concerned. When I visit schools and see a child eating a Twinkie and a Fruit Roll-Up for lunch, washing it all down with a soda pop or so-called energy drink, I wonder: How can they learn about healthy food? How can they learn about how good nutrition will help keep them physically and mentally fit? Very few schools have a curriculum for it, TV is bombarding them with enticements to eat poorly, and they are surrounded by examples of people eating with little concern for nutrition and long-term health consequences. It may be hard for us adults to change what we buy for our kids and how we eat, but we have to, for the sake of the next generation.

What has years of the modern way of food been doing to us? Let's consider a little bit of data. Since the 1960s the weight of the average American has gone up by 20 pounds, while the average height is only an inch taller. It's no wonder, because on average we've been consuming 70 pounds of sugar a year and 500 more calories a day than we did in the 1970s. That's a lot. I can't help but think of how difficult it is to burn just a few hundred during a workout.

We're eating on the run more. According to USDA figures, in 1929 we spent five times more money on eating at home than eating out. By 1955 we spent only three times as much on meals at home. Now, our expenditures for eating out are roughly equal to what we spend eating at home. As Michael Pollan,

> On average we've been consuming 70 pounds of sugar a year and 500 more calories a day than we did in the 1970s.

one of the pioneers of the healthy eating movement, likes to say, if you're getting your meal through a car window, there's a good chance it's not good for you. Snacking has also become a national pastime, particularly for adolescents. The USDA reports that four out of five adolescents have at least one snack a day, accounting for a quarter of their total calories for the day. As a result of how we eat—not taking time to have a leisurely family dinner—many doctors and nutritionists and cooks are advocating slow food. They believe we are not savoring our food, nor giving ourselves a chance to know we are satisfied, which in turn means we eat more.

Looking at satisfaction from another angle, we've learned that it's actually harder to get satisfied in a deep sense because our industrialized food simply doesn't have the taste and the aroma it once did. It doesn't provide the feast of the senses that has been an essential part of eating in the great cultures and food traditions that created the American melting pot. What our industrial food does provide is lots of sugar, fat, and salt; this is to compensate for the loss of the complex flavors our grandparents enjoyed.

According to Barry Popkin, professor of nutrition at the Carolina Population Center, three-quarters of all our foods and beverages have sugar added to them now. Popkin was interviewed by the Canadian Broadcasting Corporation's Jill Eisen, on the radio program *Ideas*.[1] Popkin says we've witnessed a food explosion: He estimates that in the early 80s we had about 10,000 to 15,000 bar codes for food products, and today we have 600,000, and most of the products are packaged food goods—junk food that makes up half of the grocery store. Just look at how big the frozen food aisle has become in the average grocery store. And our food buying and eating opportunities are not limited to grocery stores now, Popkin points out. We can get ready-to-eat food in gas stations, drug stores, and even clothing stores. Eating establishments of every stripe crowd the streetscape. With the number of eating places having increased "a thousandfold," we've become a nation of perpetual snackers, not limited to three meals a day, but something more like five or six eating events a day—often featuring sweets.

As author Michael Moss told the same program, our national sweet tooth has been nurtured steadily since the advent in the 1970s of high-fructose corn syrup, which as a liquid was much easier to introduce into many food products, in particular soda, which helped give birth to the super-size-me phenomenon and the focus on food science directed not at nutrition, but rather at tricking us into eating just one more nacho chip

---

1   I've listened to their two-part podcast "Stuffed" more than a few times. I highly recommend it. A number of the key thinkers I cite here are featured.

dipped in liquefied cheese (a near-devious combo of fat, salt, and a bit of sugar[2]).

As Michael Pollan points out in his book *In Defense of Food*:

> Since 1980, American farmers have produced an average of 600 more calories per person per day, the price of food has fallen, portion sizes have ballooned, and, predictably, we're eating a whole lot more, at least 300 more calories a day than we consumed in 1985. What kind of calories? Nearly a quarter of these additional calories come from added sugars (and most of that in the form of high-fructose corn syrup); roughly another quarter from fat (most of it in the form of soybean oil); 46 percent of them from grains (mostly refined); and the few calories left (8 percent) from fruit and vegetables. The overwhelming majority of the calories Americans have added to their diets since 1985—93 percent of them in the form of sugars, fats, and mostly refined grains—supply lots of energy but very little of anything else.

Even if we were eating the same number of calories, where these calories come from matters too, because not all calories are equal. Yes, the kind of calories matter, and the health of the bacteria in our gut matters, in complex ways that we are learning more about every

---

2   To be precise, Doritos Nacho Cheese Dip contains: Water, Vegetable Oil, Sour Cream (8%), Mature White Cheddar (5%), White Wine Vinegar, Modified Starch, Dried Skimmed Milk, Sugar, Yeast Extract, Salt, Dried Egg Yolk, Acidity Regulator (Lactic Acid), Garlic Puree, Spices, Stabilizer (Xanthan Gum), Color (Paprika Extract), Onion, Preservative (Potassium Sorbate)

day. We need fiber. We need antioxidants. We need vitamins, minerals, and things that are in whole food that we don't even understand yet, but we know instinctively are good for us. Dr. Mark Hyman, who wrote the preface for this book, likes to use the following little story to illustrate this point:

> Take a class of sixth graders. Show them a picture of one thousand calories of broccoli and one thousand calories of soda. Ask them if they have the same effect on our bodies. Their unanimous response will be "NO!" We all intuitively know that equal caloric amounts of soda and broccoli can't be the same nutritionally. But as Mark Twain said, "The problem with common sense is that it is not too common."

So let's just take a moment to consider soda, which hardly deserves the label "food." Between 1980 and 2002, average soda consumption in North America more than doubled. It tripled for teenaged boys.

||||||||||||||||||||||||||||||||||||||||||||||||||||||||||||||||||||||||||||||||||||||||||||||||||||||||||||||||||||||||||||||

FROM A HARVARD PUBLIC HEALTH FACT SHEET

SODA CONSUMPTION: STEADILY RISING SIZES AND REPERCUSSIONS

- Before the 1950s, standard soft drink sizes were 6.5 ounces. In the 1950s, soft drink companies introduced the 12-ounce can. By the 1990s, 20-ounce plastic bottles became the norm. In 2011, the 42-ounce bottle was introduced.

- In the 1970s, sugary drinks—soda, energy, sports drinks—made up about 4 percent of U.S. daily calorie intake. By 2001, it had more than doubled to 9 percent.

- From 1989 to 2008, calories from sugary beverages increased by 60 percent in children from ages 6 to 11—from 130 to 209 calories per day—and the percentage of children consuming them rose from 79 percent to 91 percent.

- On any given day, half the people in the U.S. drink sugary drinks. A quarter get at least 200 calories from sugary drinks, and 5 percent get at least 567 calories (four cans of soda).

- Sugary drinks are the top calorie source in teens' diets (226 calories per day), beating out pizza.

- A 20-year study on 120,000 men and women found that people who increased their sugary drink consumption by one 12-ounce serving per day gained more weight over time—an average of an extra pound over four years—than people who did not change their intake.

- For each 12-ounce soda children consumed each day, one study found, the odds of becoming obese increased by 60 percent during 1.5 years of follow-up.

- People who consume sugary drinks regularly—one to two cans per day or more—have a 26 percent greater risk of developing type 2 diabetes than people who rarely have such drinks.

- A 20-year study that followed 40,000 men found that those who averaged one can of a sugary drink per day had a 20 percent higher risk of having a heart attack or dying from a heart attack than men who rarely consumed sugary drinks. (A related study found the same for women.)

||||||||||||||||||||||||||||||||||||||||||||||||||||||||||||||||||||||||||||||||||||||||||||||||||||||||||||||||||||||||||||||||||||||||||||

Sure, I have a soda from time to time. I find it refreshing. But at these amounts? Ouch!

And soda is just one example of a "food" that's causing us health problems. What are the results of taking in all the empty calories we get from our subsidized fake food? A whopping bill, estimated to be in the neighborhood of $250 billion per year in diet-related health care costs.

Here's a short list of some of the conditions and diseases that doctors are now grappling with as a result of our poor eating habits:

Obesity: We've already seen how rampant this is, and it's a condition that carries a lot of what doctors call "morbidity"; that is, it's the source of many other ailments—problems with joints, depression, sexual dysfunction, just to name a few.

Diabetes: The cheap, fake food we've been consuming in vast amounts over the past couple of decades has led to a diabetes epidemic. By 2020 half of Americans will have diabetes or prediabetes. We had to change the name of adult-onset diabetes to

> **By 2020 half of Americans will have diabetes or prediabetes.**

"type 2," because so many children get the disease, and a substantial portion of those cases are diet-related. Our children are inheriting a diet that has been making us sick. What will happen to *their* children?

While diabetes is expensive enough to take care of on its own, it also complicates the treatment of almost all other health issues a person may have. And this drives up health care costs for everyone (and drives up our national debt as well). I was visiting a few doctors at Summa Health Care, a hospital system in Akron, and they told me that, while they haven't done a study to officially confirm the data, their experience tells them that the average patient who has diabetes—in addition to some other health issue like heart disease or high blood pressure—stays an average of one and a half days longer than the patient with just the original health issue. The average cost of caring for a diabetic is five times the cost of caring for an average person, according to Dr. Hyman.

High blood pressure: This condition is a major cause of strokes, and it's called "the silent killer" because it's so hard for an individual to detect on his or her own. One in every three American adults has high blood pressure, and more than 348,000 American deaths included high blood pressure as a primary or contributing cause. One in five American adults is also unaware that they have the condition.

Digestive illnesses: Issues such as gastroesophageal reflux disease and irritable bowel syndrome are on the rise. According to the American College of Gastroenterology, more than 60 million Americans experience acid reflux at least once a month and at least 15 million experience it daily. Irritable bowel syndrome is also quite common; it may affect over 15 percent of the general population. While the causes for irritable bowel syndrome are unknown, it has been found that moderating an individual's diet and limiting high fat products and dairy can lessen symptoms.

Heart disease: The connection between eating trans fats and too much sugar and getting heart disease is well established. Heart disease is the leading cause of death for both men and women. About 600,000 people die of heart disease in the U.S. every year; this is about one in every four deaths. In the United States, someone has a heart attack every 34 seconds. Each minute, someone in the United States dies from a heart disease–related event.

Cancer: The underlying causes of cancer are complex, but poor nutrition certainly seems to play a role. Each year, nearly 600,000 Americans die of cancer, and around one-third of these deaths are linked to poor diet and physical inactivity. According to the American Cancer Society, being overweight or obese can increase the risk of several cancers including colon and rectal, endometrial (uterine), esophageal, pancreatic, and breast cancers. Being overweight leads the body to produce increased amounts of estrogen and insulin, hormones that can stimulate cancer growth. A 2011 review by the British Cancer Society found that one in ten cancers may be linked to a diet that includes a high salt intake, low levels of fiber, and high intakes of red meat. Research has found that bowel cancer is less common in individuals who eat lots of fiber. And a study by the European Prospective Investigation into Cancer and Nutrition found that individuals who ate the most fiber had a 40 percent lower risk of bowel cancer than those who ate the least.

Nutrient deficiency: Intense processing of food tends to decrease the concentrations of vitamins and minerals. Food processors do "enrich" their foods by adding vitamins and minerals back in, but not in sufficient quantities to compete with the real stuff. Magnesium and potassium are two examples of nutrient deficiencies that are widespread.

According to Dr. Hyman, "By conservative standards of measurement (blood, or serum, magnesium levels), 65 percent of people admitted to the intensive care unit—and about 15 percent of the general population—have magnesium deficiency." In sufficient amounts, he says, magnesium can be "an antidote to stress," and when it is deficient, it can cause a number of adverse conditions, including inflammation, a wide variety of cramping and stiffness ailments, as well as headaches and other common maladies. As for potassium, which is mostly found in fruits and vegetables, according to the USDA's "What We Eat in America" report, "the average potassium intake of the U.S. population 2 years and older was 2640 mg per day . . . The Institute of Medicine recommendation for Adequate Intake of potassium is 4700 mg per day." Research indicates that low potassium may be associated with high blood pressure, while higher intake may reduce incidence of kidney stones and bone loss.

Mental Health Conditions: Many studies have found nutritional connections to conditions such as ADHD and bipolar disorder. Changes in diet have been found to help individuals combat the symptoms of bipolar disorder. Studies in people and rats have linked folic acid, vitamin B12, and zinc deficiency to depression. Studies have also found links between the intake of certain dietary components with the prevalence of different types of depression. Other diseases related to gluten, such as celiac disease, are also associated with mood disorders. Apart from serious disorders, common sense tells us that when we are properly fed, we are more awake and alert. We can be better students and do our jobs better. Researchers have been studying additives such as synthetic dyes, flavors, and preservatives and whether these additives contribute to hyperactivity or other symptoms in children. While the evidence suggesting that artificial additives cause ADHD is not yet extensive, some studies have shown that certain food dyes and preservatives can increase hyperactive behavior in children. One study in Britain convinced the U.K. Food Standards Agency to urge food manufacturers to remove six artificial coloring agents from food marketed to children. The authors of the study cautioned that not every child was vulnerable to artificial additives, but that there were some children who would be particularly susceptible. Another study conducted by researchers at Columbia University and Harvard University also found that removing artificial food coloring from the diets of children with ADHD would help in the treatment of their symptoms. In fact, this method was about one-third to one-half as effective as the treatment with Ritalin.

Diseases and adverse health conditions are not the end of the story, though. There are many *ripple effects* that come from poor health: decreases in the productivity and innovative capacity of our workforce; an educational "achievement gap" that puts our children near the bottom of developed nations in math and reading because kids can't learn on a sugary junk food diet; a hampered ability to compete economically; and a diversion of time and effort and ingenuity to address these preventable diseases that could be focused on other big problems we have to tackle, such as creating a new and dynamic education system, increasing innovation and entrepreneurism in our national economy, or improving our environment. Given all of this it seems obvious to me that . . . it's the food, stupid!

We need to be eating a different mix of foods, and we may need some supplements to make up for deficiencies in the nutrient makeup of modern foods. And I'm not talking here about individuals going on diets. Diets are next to impossible to maintain—particularly in a food environment where we are surrounded by so much of the wrong stuff that is so enticing to our raw animal instincts for survival. We need to realign our national food supply (over a period of time, but steadily), so that it's more in line with what will keep us healthy and avoid costly diseases.

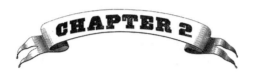

OUR BROKEN ENVIRONMENT

High levels of pesticides sprayed on our crops, run-offs from heavily fertilized fields, and the practices of factory farming are damaging the delicate ecosystem that surrounds our food production.

Mother Nature bats last, and she always bats a thousand.

—ROBERT K. WATSON

When I was about ten years old, I found a very small clearing under some trees way back behind our house. I decided it would be a perfect place to build a fort. I ran back to the house and asked my mother if it would be okay with her, and she said fine. The ground was covered with several years' worth of old dead leaves, so I decided to clear them out using a snow shovel. I was digging vigorously when a swarm of bees came out of the pile. I was stung several times right away, and as I ran back to the house screaming and crying, I was stung many times more. By the time I reached my house, I had been stung about 15 times. Man, that hurt . . . for days.

All this is to say, I have no reason to love bees. In fact, I'm still a little spooked by them when they're buzzing near me. But I do love honey, and I also think the whole process of pollination is simply one of the most magical processes on God's green earth. Certain plants require insects to visit them and spread their pollen in order to flourish. Then the bees produce honey and interestingly its taste is influenced by the type of plants the bees pollinate. I will never stop being impressed by this.

Sadly, as you will see later in this chapter, bees are losing out in the fight for survival—and it may well have something to do with our high-intensity industrial agriculture methods, which don't seem to be in sync with Mother Nature. It's not only our personal health that is affected by our modern way of food; it is also the health of the earth, which is ultimately about the health of every living creature on the planet.

American farming has changed rapidly in the last several decades. Many of the small- and medium-scale farms have disappeared. Farms are now giant productions that have a laser focus on increased productivity and efficiency. They strive for this through the use of new technology and farming practices, and in fact, modern farms have become much more "efficient." Since 1960, milk production has doubled, meat production has tripled, and egg production has quadrupled. The raising of livestock

> In 1920, a chicken took approximately 16 weeks to reach 2.2 pounds. Now they can reach 5 pounds in 7 weeks.

has also been manipulated to become much faster. As an example, in 1920, a chicken took approximately 16 weeks to reach 2.2 pounds. Now they can reach 5 pounds in 7 weeks.

In a report from Food & Water Watch, a group that works to ensure the safety and accessibility of the food, fish, and water we consume, it was stated that the total number of livestock on the largest factory farms rose by more than one-fifth between 2002 and 2007. What's more:

- The number of livestock units on factory farms rose 21.2 percent from 23.8 million in 2002 to 28.8 million in 2007.

- Dairy cows on factory farms have nearly doubled. The number of dairy cows rose 93.4 percent from 2.5 million cows in 1997 to 4.9 million in 2007.

- Broiler chickens on the largest factory farms have nearly doubled to one billion.

- Factory farm operations (where there are at least 500 or more head of cattle) make up 47.7 percent of the total cattle inventory; in 1999, the figure was 38 percent.

And these increases don't just apply to raising animals. Average corn yields have gone up by approximately 500 percent since the beginning of the 20th century. In the 1920s they averaged around 25 bushels per acre farmed, but in the past few years, that has gone up to more than 150 bushels per acre! While the increase in barley production hasn't been nearly as dramatic, we are still producing nearly 70 bushels per acre now as opposed to the average of 20 bushels in the 1920s.

So what does this mean for the health of our planet— and ourselves?

Thanks to the sophisticated engineering methods that resulted in "concentrated animal feeding operations," or CAFOs, which can contain hundreds of thousands of animals, we've seen a terrible impact on the environments surrounding these operations.

Because these lots are packed with animals, the living conditions are very unhealthy. Disease is rampant, which leads to the use of antibiotics. In addition, these factory farming operations use hormones to promote growth in cattle and sheep. (Hormone use is banned by the USDA in animals other than cattle and sheep.) According to an estimate in *Science News,* in an article by Janet Raloff, more than 80 percent of cattle in America are given hormones to stimulate more rapid growth. Raloff writes:

> Many cattle are fed the same muscle-building androgens—usually testosterone surrogates—that some athletes consume. Other animals receive estrogens, the primary female sex hormones, or progestins, semiandrogenic agents that shut down a female's estrus cycle. Progestins fuel meat-building by freeing up

resources that would have gone into the reproductive cycle . . . A substantial portion of the hormones literally passes through the cattle into their feces and ends up in the environment, where it can get into other food and drinking water.

These antibiotics and hormones not only end up in our food and milk, they have also been detected in significant amounts in groundwater and waterways adjacent to feedlots. Raloff cites a study by Louis J. Guillette, Jr., of the University of Florida and Ana M. Soto of Tufts University School of Medicine in Boston that investigated hormones in runoff from feedlots in Nebraska and their effect on fish populations. Male fathead minnows downstream had a significantly reduced testis size, which Guillette said appears to explain why they also produced less testosterone than males upstream. He also found that the heads of these fathead minnows were smaller, which he thinks is related to the hormonal intake, since testosterone helps determine skull size.

We are lacing our water with pharmaceuticals. This raises concerns about creating an increased resistance to antibiotics through overexposure. I will discuss antibiotics and hormones more in chapter 6, when I talk about campaigns under way to rethink how we get our food. But for now, let's consider some of the other ways that our food system is harming the earth and our health.

The CAFOs and large factory farms are big polluters, causing more problems than just those of increases in antibiotics and hormones. They produce an estimated 500 million to 1 billion tons of manure annually. Just so you can see how substantial this is, consider that municipal wastewater treatment plants annually treat 18 million tons of human fecal material. The animal waste contains high levels of nitrates and phosphorus; pathogens, including bacteria; and metals such as copper or arsenic. And this dangerous combo is usually stored with minimal or no treatment in waste lagoons before being applied to cropland as fertilizer. In the event of storms or due to poor management, these animal wastes can wash away

> **Factory farms produce an estimated 500 million to I billion tons of manure annually.**

from uncovered manure piles or leak from waste lagoons into groundwater. The high levels of nitrates in animal wastes have been linked to health problems, including miscarriages, cancer, and gastrointestinal problems.

The EPA National Water Quality Inventory reported that agriculture—both crops and livestock—is the leading source of water quality impairment on rivers and lakes. Within these findings, 29 states identified livestock feeding operations as a source of water impairments. An EPA risk assessment report found that drinking-water sources for an estimated 43 percent of the U.S. population have suffered some level of pathogen contamination associated with CAFOs. So, almost 60 percent of our states are hurt by this current setup, and almost half of our population. This is not some isolated incident or random event, as some would want you to believe. It is systemic, serious, and must be addressed soon.

In addition, in a briefing on climate change, the EPA notes that globally, the agriculture sector is the largest producer of methane, and "Pound for pound, the comparative impact of methane on climate change is over 20 times greater than carbon dioxide over a 100-year period." The air pollution from manure—which produces a prodigious stink in high-production areas—may be the source of many a joke, but it's clear that the levels of methane gas we're producing in our livestock operations is unsustainable. Scott Faber, senior vice president of government affairs for the Environmental Working Group, also notes that the fertilizer and manure we're spreading on fields releases nitrous oxide into the air, and when land is cleared for crop production, soil carbon is released. Dietary change is linked to climate change. We live in an interconnected world.

The big "advance" to increase production in industrial food farming is the introduction of genetically modified seeds, also called genetically engineered (GE) seeds. These seeds are designed to be resistant to a variety of substances. For example, seed could be modified to resist a certain herbicide so a field could be sprayed to get rid of weeds but not kill the crop. A practice like this increases the yield and therefore profits. Other seeds might be designed to stave off certain insects, which means less money spent on herbicides and pesticides, meaning lower overhead and higher profits, and less herbicide. Good, right?

Enter Mother Nature, the ultimate adapter! After several years of planting GE seeds like this, the weeds adapted and so did insects like the Western corn rootworm, which is corn's nemesis. The farmers had a natural response: spray *heavier doses* of herbicides and pesticides to kill the weeds and the pests. And as the weed resistance grew over the last decade, herbicide use skyrocketed. Food & Water Watch has reported a total on-farm herbicide increase of 26 percent between 2001 and 2010. Ouch!

Roundup is the industry-leading herbicide from Monsanto, the $12 billion chemical giant. An April 2014 report from the Arctic University of Norway found "extreme levels" of Roundup in GE soy. The University of Norway researchers used Monsanto's own definition of what "extreme levels" were for Roundup per kilogram. In 1999 they said 5.6 milligrams per kilo of plant weight was "extreme." The study found high levels of Roundup on 70 percent of the GE soy plants they looked at in Iowa, with an average of 9 milligrams of Roundup per kilo, close to double Monsanto's own definition. I can picture the waiter in the fancy, white-tableclothed restaurant now: "Would you like some soy with your Roundup, sir?"

A German-led study, published in the *Journal of Environmental & Analytical Toxicology*, also found high levels of glyphosate (the active ingredient in Roundup) in the urine of dairy cows—and people. These levels of glyphosate in both humans and animals might adversely affect the health of the entire population.

These high levels of pesticides are damaging the delicate ecosystem that surrounds our food production. We are seeing changes in populations of insects and animals who are exposed to heavy concentrations of these chemicals. For example, Factory-Farming.com has published a lot of information on what is called "Colony Collapse Disorder" (CCD).

Bees lose colonies every winter; it's a natural process. But last year they lost 800,000 colonies, or 31 percent of the total. This is up from 22 percent the previous year, and the number has been growing steadily since 2006.

While nobody seems to know exactly why this is happening, it's a matter of great concern because the USDA says that $20 billion worth of annual harvests depend on bee pollination. Many crops, like apricots, peaches, apples, and almonds, heavily depend on bee pollination.

> **$20 billion worth of annual harvests depend on bee pollination.**

While it hasn't been proven and there are many potential factors leading to the decrease in honey bees, scientists suspect there is a correlation between CCD and the heavy use of pesticides, especially neonicotinoids, which are nicotine based. I'm not even sure how to pronounce that word, but whatever it is, it's used heavily in Midwestern corn states, which is where many beekeepers keep their hives in the summertime. Hmm. Interestingly, Factory-Farming.com has reported that Europe is preparing to ban this substance until scientists can figure out what its effect on the bee population is. (Meanwhile, a group of engineers at Harvard are working to develop "robobees" that could be digital pollinators once we've killed off all the real bees. Is this really what we have our best minds working on?)

Another species getting killed off is bats. The decrease in population started in the Northeast with bats contracting what scientists call white-nose syndrome (because a white fungus covers the bat's nose and wings). It's now spreading to bats in the South as far down as North Carolina and Tennessee. Why is this important? A single bat can eat between 600 and 1,000 mosquitoes an hour. If bats get killed off, insect populations will increase. More bugs mean more pesticides. More pesticides mean more Roundup on our food and potentially fewer bees and reductions in crops that rely on bee pollination. It's one vicious circle after another.

These are just two examples of many—the biodiversity of our environment is suffering greatly under our current system.

Another area of concern is pesticide and fertilizer runoff in our waterways. Common sense tells us that the oil-based chemicals spread over our food must eventually get into our aquifers, rivers, lakes, and oceans. In the latest National Water Quality Inventory, the Environmental Protection Agency found that 40 percent of the surveyed rivers and lakes were not clean enough for fishing or swimming! What a huge blow to our environment and our quality of life. There are many places in Ohio where fishing, boating, and swimming are major forms of family entertainment and recreation (and for fisherman, a contribution to feeding their families).

Many of the fertilizers used in farming contain nitrogen, and only about 30 to 50 percent reaches the plant, according to a 2012 study in the *Plant Biotechnology Journal*. The rest is washed away into the local ecosystem. As Michael Pollan writes in *The Omnivore's Dilemma*, "The flood of synthetic nitrogen has fertilized not just the farm fields but the forests and the oceans too . . . [They] flow down the Mississippi into the Gulf of Mexico, where their deadly fertility poisons the marine ecosystem. The nitrogen tide stimulates the wild growth of algae, and the algae smother the fish, creating a 'hypoxic,' or dead, zone as big as the state of New Jersey—and still growing."

Algae blooms are also making their way into the Great Lakes, including the record-setting 5,000-kilometer algae bloom in Lake Erie in 2011. These are not only terrible for biodiversity and the environment; they are huge blows to local economies that rely on tourism and fishing as major engines of economic development. Other dead zones include the Florida Everglades and the Chesapeake Bay.

In Midwestern states, millions of dollars are spent on water treatment plants to remove agricultural chemicals. None of these costs are borne by our food suppliers. If they were, they would find their way into the price of food, and we would rebel. But the taxpayers in these local areas are certainly footing the bill for trying to reverse the damage of the current system. There is an ever-growing cost associated with our agriculture practices, and our environment continues to be degraded.

The damage isn't just limited to the short term, either. In the long term, the practices used by corporate farms could actually create problems for growing crops, and thus would require more technological intervention (maybe those Harvard engineers can start on "robo-dirt" once they're done with the bees). Modern farming practices, for example, cause dangerous amounts of soil erosion. Agricultural practices dramatically increase the rate of erosion. Tilling land removes a protective layer of topsoil that helps hold soil together. A 2007 USDA Natural Resources Conservation Service report found that the rate of soil erosion averaged 5.2 tons per acre per year. This is apparently a reassuring estimate, because 5 tons per acre per year is considered a "sustainable" loss. However, an Environmental Working Group report challenged the USDA findings, showing evidence that the rate of soil erosion is much higher. Recent storms in Iowa have triggered soil losses of 64 tons of soil per acre, 12 times greater than the federal government's reported average. In addition, researchers found that the rate of soil loss across Iowa was twice the sustainable rate estimated by the USDA.

Soil erosion is a major concern for our world food supply. Once enough soil is removed, the land becomes unable to sustain crops. One study estimates that over the past 40 years, 30 percent of the world's arable land has become unproductive as a result of erosion!

Naturally, then, there is increasing effort to plow more land to increase crop yields—both to feed us and to feed the herds of animals in these farms. These actions don't just clear land for food, they negatively impact biodiversity. For example, they take out native plants like milkweed that provide nectar for many species. A 2012 study published in the journal *Insect Conservation and Diversity* (thank heaven such journals exist) found that Iowa has lost almost 60 percent of its milkweed, and another in *Crop Protection* found a 90 percent reduction from 1999 to 2009.

The massively efficient industrial food we've created is massively profitable to a few who are in charge of it, but it's a blunt instrument that does not take into account the delicacy of our ecosystem and the connections between plants, animals, humans, air, water, and soil. It treats the earth and its creatures as if they were machines. And, as we have seen, the machine is breaking down.

Whether you are Republican, Democrat, Independent, Tea Party, Libertarian, what have you, how can you advocate for a system that is ruining the very land, air, and water we rely on?

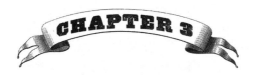

THE POWER OF GOVERNMENT AND BIG BUSINESS

The large corporations at the heart of the current food system, supported by our government, dictate what's available to eat at what price. If it's not working for you, you need to fight back.

> *The history of agriculture policy in the United States is one of increasing concentration and consolidation, with big driving out small in the name of efficiency.*
>
> —MARION NESTLE

We are all connected to many different systems that support life. In addition to our social systems—family, community, church, and so on—there are huge national and international systems that undergird our life. And they often go unnoticed as we go about our day. They're so much a part of us, they're like the water a fish swims in. You flick on a light switch or plug in your phone to charge it, and you're relying on our energy system. Your daughter goes to school, and you're relying on a vast network that makes up our education system. You drive to the airport and fly your family to see Grandma, and you're relying on our transportation system. You get sick, you rely on the health care system. You spend money, it's the banking system. You go to the bathroom . . . okay, you get the picture.

We put these systems together, for the most part, with the best of intentions. We're trying to create a good life. You know—life, liberty, and the pursuit of happiness. But sometimes a system goes bad. How do we know? Because the outcome is not a happy one. That's what's happening with the food system. As I've made clear already, the food system is not achieving its aim of fostering our health and well-being and that of our environment. I'm sorry. It's just not. End of story. I'm not going to debate that anymore.

But then you have to figure out what to do about a system gone bad. That's a tough one. There's a lot we can do as individuals to improve how we collectively manage our food system, but before we do that, we have to understand what got us to where we are, and what's keeping us here.

II

FULL DISCLOSURE

As I talk about lobbying and fundraising and its impact on the political system, it is important for you to know that I too have taken money from a few of the organizations that are involved in the food industry, primarily the sugar industry. But as you can tell from the fact that I have written this book and will promote the ideas in it in a very public way, campaign contributions do not influence the way I think or the way I vote. If they did, I would not talk about these issues. But through the course of my career in Congress, I work with groups that may agree with my position on some very important issues and disagree on some others. For example, we may see eye-to-eye on trade issues but disagree on certain kinds of subsidies. These organizations have chosen to support my campaign fund, and I appreciate their help, as every politician needs money to run for reelection. But let me say clearly that no campaign donation has ever led me to compromise my beliefs or my votes. I have never let money influence my decision-making and I never will. I will speak my mind and let the chips fall as they may. As an aside, I am one of only a handful of members who support publicly financed campaigns. It is the surest way to clean up our broken system and get money out of politics.

IIIIIIIIIIIIIIIIIIIIIIIIIIIIIIIIIIIIIIIIIIIIIIIIIIIIIIIIIIIIIIIIIIIIIIIIIIIIIIIIIIIIIIIIIIIIIIIIIIIIIIIIIIIIIIIIIIIIIIIIIIII

One of the major developments that brought us to this sorry state of affairs, Michael Pollan explains, was change in agricultural policy, which began under President Richard Nixon in the 1970s. In order to fight food price inflation, we began rewarding farmers to grow *more* food, whereas previous policies tried to support food prices by reducing supply; for example, by idling land. This helped the farmers rather than looking out for the consumers. But with this change, Pollan says, the federal government gave growers incentives to *overproduce.*

This policy kept prices down for consumers, all right, but as I've learned the hard way in my last 14 years in government, there are always unintended consequences for any policy we enact. The overproduction rippled throughout the system and we ended up with what we have now. There's a lot more grain, and that cheap grain in the form of corn became cheap corn sweetener, available to sweeten everything imaginable. The increased supply of grain was one factor that caused us to end up with the feedlot meat system, which gives us meat filled with hormones and antibiotics instead of nature's original grass-fed beef. We subsidized the grain-based foods—processed foods and lower quality meat from big producers, essentially—making them cheap, while providing almost no support for fruits and vegetables. The story goes on from there, but you get the picture. All those cheap calories made their way to the American waistline, and taught a whole generation of kids how to eat too much, and poorly.

Marion Nestle, author of *Food Politics* and *Eat, Drink, Vote*, is a public health nutritionist and professor at New York University. Like Pollan, she points out that we've ended up with a system that "is very efficient and provides an overabundance of foods from which to choose at relatively low cost," but it seems to revolve around one principle: to produce calories as cheaply as possible.

So let's dive a little deeper into this system that keeps us in this sad state of affairs, starting with the farm bill, which, from 1995 to 2012, allotted $292 billion of our tax money to subsidize our broken farm program. Yes, I said

> From 1995 to 2012, the farm bill has allotted $292 billion of our tax money to subsidize our broken farm program.

292 BILLION DOLLARS. That's nine zeros. Even in Washington, DC, that is a boatload of money. I'm guessing you have no desire to read the 959 pages of the farm bill that passed in 2014, so let me tell you just a little bit about it—including the problems that I found with it.

The "farm bill" is the shorthand name for a massive piece of legislation that Congress enacts about every five years. It authorizes the federal government to spend money on dozens of programs that are intended to provide us with a working food system while conserving land and protecting, maintaining, and improving the soil, water, and air that supply us with the food. The farm bill is not the only piece of legislation that governs agriculture, but it is by far the largest and most significant. The first farm bill was enacted in 1933 in response to the economic depression and the dust bowl in that era. Its goal was to keep our farmers in business while also encouraging conservation. Subsidies for key commodities such as corn and wheat have continued to rise in farm bill after farm bill over the decades; however, these subsidies have not been in line with the original intention of keeping struggling farmers in business. They now disproportionately benefit the richest of the farmers and the big agricultural companies that supply these farmers.

Over the years, the farm bill added other elements. The 1973 bill provided nutrition assistance in the form of food stamps (now called the Supplemental Nutrition Assistance Program, or SNAP). The 1985 bill was notable for including new conservation laws; the 1990 bill included organic agriculture for the first time; the 1996 bill included the Fund for Rural America, to increase USDA research into innovations in farming (thank you, Bill Clinton); and the 2008 farm bill included provisions to promote local food systems, including the Farmers Market Promotion Program.

The farm bill began with good intentions—to save our farmers and our food supply during the Great Depression. And many good programs have been enacted over the years, but in general, I feel the legislation has strayed from the fundamentals:

To ensure a food system that supports our farmers' work in providing healthy, nutritional food while conserving our land and environment

As I have made clear, we are failing to do this. So, the kind of farm bill and overall food legislative program I want to see would realign priorities and increase funding for:

- Sustainable regional and urban agriculture systems

- Conservation and environmental protection

- Non-genetically modified food and organically grown food

- Actions that to encourage complete transparency concerning ingredients and processes
- Beginning farmers
- Vegetable and fruit growing
- Innovation research and agricultural extension programs
- Nutrition education from K–12 to college to medical school

(I might add that I like the idea that Michael Pollan shared with me of having a national food policy advisor as a senior official in the White House. We have a national security advisor. "Isn't our food supply just as important to our well-being as defense?" he asks. Makes sense to me. Michelle's Obama's tireless work in bringing nutrition issues to the forefront of the national conversation is the kind of leadership we are going to need on this issue in all future administrations. The appointment of Sam Kass as Senior Policy Advisor for Nutrition Policy has also been a good step toward a higher-level administration position. This White House has us off to a great start.)

The bill that passed Congress this year, known formally as the Agricultural Act of 2014, did not come close to initiating the kind of reform that I would like to see, given the fact that our food system is yielding so many unhealthy outcomes. It took no steps to decrease the levels of antibiotics and hormones in our meat and poultry. It carried on the gross subsidies (now called crop insurance) to large-scale commercial agriculture, while offering a paltry sum for sustainable and regional specialty farmers. And when I refer to sustainable and regional farms, I'm not just talking about "certified organic." Many farmers have an approach that is similar to organic, but getting the certification is so time-consuming and costly that it isn't worth the trouble

While 98 percent of farms are family-owned operations, only a small percentage receive agricultural subsidies. Over

> While 98 percent of farms are family-owned operations, only a small percentage receive agricultural subsidies. Over the last ten years, 62 percent of farms collected no subsidy.

the last ten years, 62 percent of farms collected no subsidy at all. Emerging, innovative local farmers do not get a leg up. The already entrenched farmers get the "help." For all these reasons, I voted against the bill, and am working now to correct problems with it and pave the way for a farm bill that people interested in good nutrition and a sound environment can get behind. (For those interested in farm bill reform, the Environmental Working Group [www.ewg.org] provides excellent information on how the money is spent now, and a vision for how it could be better spent.)

One of the reasons it's so hard to change policy is the power of lobbyists sent to DC on behalf of these corporate interests. For a member of Congress, being lobbied is a daily activity, whether it's someone at the grocery store or dry cleaners at home telling you how they feel about the issue they feel most passionate about, or a more formal sit-down in a congressional office in Washington, DC. Most of the formal meetings are pretty cordial, with people from Ohio who belong to an organization asking for my support on a particular issue. On occasion, my whole day is filled with sit-downs. I'm happy to do it. The day I start complaining about this is the day I should retire, because the best part about our democracy is that people can walk into their congressperson's office and state their views.

Sometimes, however, these meetings can get uncomfortable. Like earlier this year when I had to meet with the Ohio Farm Bureau. It was uneasy because just weeks before I had voted against a compromise farm bill that, while making a number of improvements, simply did not go far enough. The Farm Bureau felt I should have supported it. Agriculture is the top industry in Ohio. Unfortunately, according to the Centers for Disease Control and Prevention, 10 percent of adults in Ohio have diabetes (and another 16 states are as bad or worse), and it's estimated that over 500,000 adults in Ohio have been told by doctors that they have prediabetes, while a much larger number have the condition but are undiagnosed. I firmly believe the high incidence is largely due to our current food system, and it's worth remembering that treating the people suffering from this condition costs five times more than the average person.

The Farm Bureau folks were friendly, but we had a frank exchange about why I voted against the bill. I really like these people. I read their magazine every month, and I note that they have more and more articles about smaller farms. So, I think it's fair for me to point out when I think we can do better. If we can provide a strong alternative—a thoughtful, balanced agenda—in my estimation the majority of farm bureau members would see it as in their best interest for the future and support it.

During our discussion, I pointed out some initiatives outside of the farm bill that I thought needed attention, such as the fact that the current Congress is trying to limit transparency by rejecting labeling and warnings that would let consumers know what's in the food they're buying, what country it is from, and how it was produced. And these standards for GMO and country-of-origin label-

> Congress is trying to limit transparency by rejecting labeling and warnings that would let consumers know what is in the food they're buying and how it was produced.

ing need to be national ones. A state-by-state approach would be a nightmare for businesses to deal with, as many of them ship products to many different states. But we do need transparency for the consumer. Most farmers agree with this. In fact, just this past summer the corn and soy associations in Ohio voiced their support for labeling. Sadly, some very powerful interests aren't on the same page.

You may fairly ask, "Is this food genetically engineered?"

The big industry folks say it's none of your business. They have adopted the stance my Italian grandmother used to take with my brother and me when we were eating at her dinner table and acting up. She would say in her local Italian dialect, *"Sta zitta. Mangia."* It translates into "Shut up and eat!"

If we ask the food industry, What's in this food?

Shut up and eat!

Is it genetically engineered?

Shut up and eat!

If my children eat more than a small amount, will they get diabetes?

Shut up and eat!

If my diet relies on this processed food, will I get heart disease?

Shut up and eat!

I could take this from my grandmother, who was feeding us homegrown veggies from the garden and carefully prepared homemade meals. But I will not accept this attitude from monopolists who consistently try to hide what they're doing, including what political contributions they're making to keep the current system intact. The companies use perfectly legal means that make it difficult for you and me to trace the sources of contributions, but just because it's legal doesn't mean it's praiseworthy.

||||||||||||||||||||||||||||||||||||||||||||||||||||||||||||||||||||||||||||||||||||||||||||||||||||||||||||||||||||||

POLITICAL PRESSURE BY INDUSTRY

Wheeling and dealing by big corporations is one of the things that keeps the farm bill skewed. According to the Center for Responsive Politics, a nonprofit watchdog on federal lobbying dollars:

- 325 organizations and individuals registered as lobbyists in 2013 to work on the Senate farm bill.

- $111.5 million was spent by agricultural industries in lobbying during that time period; lobbying in the agriculture sector totaled nearly $150 million in 2013.

One example of the strength of the corporate lobbying dollar is the Corn Refiners Association (CRA), a trade association that is made up of six giant corporations, including Cargill and Archer Daniels Midland. In recent years, the CRA has been spending tons of money to promote a positive image for high-fructose corn syrup. Between 2000 and 2013, the CRA spent approximately $5.2 million in federal lobbying. It was also revealed that the CRA spent more than $30 million on a private PR campaign, including $10 million to fund a four-year research project by a cardiologist that disputed the contention that there are any negative health consequences from corn-based sweeteners!

Separately from the CRA, Archer Daniels Midland spent $1.79 million on federal lobbying on Agricultural Services issues, which the company listed as "issues related to food, feed, and renewable fuel." Its CRA partner Cargill spent $1.4 million in 2013 lobbying on crop production and processing issues, with specific issues listed as "poultry processing, partially hydrogenated vegetable oil rulemaking, food labeling and claims, food additive regulations, pathogen regulation, antibiotics."

Food and beverage companies also spend heavily to influence legislators, spending $185 million on federal lobbying between 2009 and 2013.

The effort to maintain the status quo through influence doesn't stop at our borders. In 2003, when the World Health Organization published dietary guidelines suggesting that no more than 10 percent of an adult's daily calories should come from "free" sugars (those added to food, as well as natural sugars in honey, syrup, and fruit juice), the U.S. Sugar Association pressed the federal government to withdraw funding for the WHO if the organization did not modify its recommendations. Fortunately, the WHO did not buckle from this kind of pressure, and in 2014, has recommended cutting the level to 5 percent.

One of the people representing corporate interests called my office after I voted against the farm bill. My staff told me how disappointed this group was with my vote. I told my legislative director to call him back and tell him why I voted against it and explain my plan for shifting the food system in America.

Their response: "We can't afford that."

Really?

Let me get this straight, we can afford to give this small, elite group of businesses a blatant handout, while we screw (er, I mean neglect) the small- and medium-scale farmer and perpetuate a system that causes half of our population to have either diabetes or prediabetes? That's okay?

At the time the farm bill was being debated, the renowned economist Joseph Stiglitz wrote a post on *The New York Times'* Opinionator Blog, called the "Insanity of Our Food Policy." I was glad to see an economist who could see the absurdity of what we're doing, and I thought he summed up nicely what's wrong:

> American food policy has long been rife with head-scratching illogic. We spend billions every year on farm subsidies, many of which help wealthy commercial operations to plant more crops than we need . . . As small numbers of Americans have grown extremely wealthy, their political power has also ballooned to a disproportionate size. Small, powerful interests—in this case, wealthy commercial farmers—help create market-skewing public policies that benefit

only themselves, appropriating a larger slice of the nation's economic pie.

This is what we are up against. The will of a secretive, entrenched monopoly is pitted against the will of America's parents—and the farmers who want to do right by them. I'm placing my bet with the moms, dads, and the next generation of Americans who want transparency, openness, and fresh, tasty, local, healthy food.

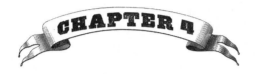

COSTS AND ACCESS

Our food system is technologically efficient but socially deficient. It is not delivering healthy, affordable food to large numbers of our citizens, in either the cities or the countryside.

> *Equal access to healthy, affordable food should be a civil right—every bit as important as access to clean air, clean water, or the right to vote.*
>
> —WILL ALLEN

The real food revolution has been driven, in large part, by people living in the more affluent zip codes in America—though not exclusively. It's time for this revolution to spread to all our citizens. In many of our cities, food deserts abound where for miles on end families with no real means of transportation have zero access to fresh, healthy food. The corner store is filled with junk food, soda, and processed ready-to-eat meals that all too often our fellow citizens eat as breakfast, lunch, or dinner. This same population has very high rates of diabetes. Our country needs a strategy to help our inner cities move from places of consumption of crappy food to places of production of good food.

The lack of access to healthy food is a problem that impacts not only the physical health of a community's residents, but also the economic and social health of the community altogether. Poverty and poor nutrition are intertwined. According to a University of North Carolina study, communities with limited access to healthy foods tend to be places with "higher poverty rates, lower median incomes, higher numbers of convenience and fast food stores per capita, more households without access to a vehicle, and larger minority populations." While a lack of fresh food may not cause poverty, it certainly makes it more difficult to rise out of poverty if you're not being given access to good nutrition.

Grocery stores and fresh food retailers provide a commercial hub that allows neighborhoods to grow, creating jobs and fostering local economies. A Food Trust report sums it up: "Access to healthy food promotes healthy local economies, healthy neighborhoods, and healthy people."

The USDA reported in 2009 that 23.5 million people lack access to a supermarket within a mile of their home, and a multistate study found that low-income areas had half as many supermarkets as wealthy areas. In predominantly white neighborhoods, there were four times as many supermarkets compared to predominantly black ones. A similar study reported that 8 percent of African Americans live in an area with a supermarket, compared to 31 percent of whites. Low-income areas tend to have a greater number of convenience stores (30 percent more than middle-income areas), which lack healthy and fresh items. A 2005 study called "The Availability and Cost of Healthier Food Alternatives" found that uniformly smaller grocery store/convenience stores lack whole-grain products, low-fat cheeses, and low-fat ground meats.

> **The USDA reported in 2009 that 23.5 million people lack access to a supermarket within a mile of their home, and a multistate study found that low-income areas had half as many supermarkets as wealthy areas.**

Put simply, people in economically disadvantaged areas are deprived of good food, and this is affecting their health. Here are a few facts to consider:

- In Albany, New York, 80 percent of nonwhite residents cannot find low-fat milk or high-fiber bread in their neighborhoods.

- In Baltimore, 46 percent of lower-income neighborhoods have limited access to healthy food compared to 13 percent of higher-income neighborhoods.

- In California, obesity and diabetes rates are 20 percent higher for those living in the least healthy food environments.

- In Chicago and Detroit, it was found that residents who live farther from grocery stores than from convenience stores and fast food restaurants have significantly higher rates of premature death from diabetes.

- A statistical modeling study estimated that adding a new grocery store to a low-income neighborhood in Indianapolis would lead to a three-pound weight decrease among its residents.

Even if you can get access to better food, food cost is a big factor in healthy eating choices. USDA researchers found that the cost of the healthier food deterred people from choosing those foods, using a market-basket survey that compared the USDA Thrifty Food Plan basket versus a healthier market basket. The USDA Thrifty Food Plan is a meal plan for a family of four for a diet that meets the minimum recommendations of the 1995 dietary guidelines. It found that for a two-week shopping list, the average Thrifty Food Plan market basket was $194, and the healthier market basket was $230, mainly because of the higher costs of whole grains and lean meats. The higher-costing healthier basket is equal to 35 to 40 percent of low-income consumers' food budgets of $2,410 a year.

> For a two-week shopping list, the average Thrifty Food Plan market basket was $194, and the healthier market basket was $230.

|||||||||||||||||||||||||||||||||||||||||||||||||||||||||||||||||||||||||||||||||||||||||||||||||||||||||||

DOES FAST FOOD REALLY COST LESS?

I feel strongly that the price gap between real, healthy food and fake food with lower nutritional value needs to shrink. Of course, it's also the case that food marketers are fooling people into thinking they are getting bargains when they go out for a fast food meal or buy sugary cereal that is marked down. If you actually buy fresh food, and take a little bit of time to prepare it, the cost will almost always be lower than feeding your family at a fast food restaurant. To a certain extent, we are paying for convenience at the cost of our health. But is it more convenient if we have to give children insulin shots every day? Is it more convenient to end up with a generation that is the first to live shorter lives than their parents? Is it more convenient if young people today need more health care when they reach their productive working years?

|||||||||||||||||||||||||||||||||||||||||||||||||||||||||||||||||||||||||||||||||||||||||||||||||||||||||||

Fruits and vegetables have also become more expensive for everyone over the years, because our subsidy system puts a little too much emphasis on grain production and provides little assistance to specialty crop farmers. (Including fruits and vegetables under crop insurance in the most recent farm bill is a step in the right direction.)

Marion Nestle notes in her Food Politics blog: "The Department of Commerce reports that the indexed price of fresh fruits and vegetables has increased by 40% since 1980, whereas the indexed price of sodas has declined by about 30%. Fast food, snacks, and sodas are cheap. Fruits and vegetables are not. Without access to healthful foods, people cannot eat healthfully."

Price discrepancies build favoritism toward bad, cheap food—the kind you see heavily advertised in grocery store flyers.

That's just considering the cost of fruits and vegetables grown by conventional methods. As is well-known, the costs of organic fruits and vegetables (and those that are organic for all intents and purposes but without the certification) tend to be much higher today (although bargains can be had at many farmers' markets). Comprehensive nationwide data is hard to come by, but in early 2011 a hearty and highly motivated group of Colby College students surveyed prices for organic and nonorganic items at five grocery stores in Waterville, Maine. Here were the results of what they found for produce:

Produce	Nonorganic	Organic	Price difference
Romaine Lettuce	$1.78/head	$3.54/head	99%
Carrots	$0.77/lb.	$1.51/lb.	96%
Bananas	$0.57/lb.	$0.89/lb.	56%
Tomatoes	$2.82/lb.	$4.05/lb.	44%
Red Peppers	$2.76/lb.	$5.89/lb.	113%
Yellow Onions	$0.93/lb.	$1.57/lb.	69%
Apples	$1.57/lb.	$2.34/lb.	49%

The Maine Organic Farmers and Gardeners Association did find that prices for produce at farmers' markets tended to be lower, given the economies of direct selling (organic lettuce sold for 18 percent less than organic lettuce in the supermarket, for example). Nevertheless, if this is the kind of food we want to promote for our own health and the health of the planet, the cost is still too high.

It's also the case that while our fruits and vegetables have been going up in price, they have been decreasing in nutritional quality due to depletion of soil quality from high-intensity agriculture methods—which emphasize quantity over quality—according to several authorities both here and in the United Kingdom. In its EarthTalk blog, *Scientific American* estimated that to get the same amount of vitamin A our grandparents derived from one orange, we would need to eat eight. We are paying more money for less nutrition.

It would be easy to think that city dwellers

> **To get the same amount of vitamin A our grandparents derived from one orange, we would need to eat eight.**
>
> —EARTHTALK, *SCIENTIFIC AMERICAN*

are the only ones who experience high prices and availability problems for fresh food, since rural people are closer to the source, but that is sadly not true. There are many "rural food deserts," where all residents live more than ten miles from a supermarket or supercenter. A nationwide analysis found that there are 418 rural food desert counties—20 percent of all rural counties in the U.S. In Mississippi, the state with the highest obesity rate in the country (35.4 percent of adults), over 70 percent of food stamp–eligible households travel more than 30 miles to reach a supermarket. The lack of supermarkets and access to fresh food correspond to the likelihood of fresh food consumption. In rural Mississippi, residents in food desert counties are 23 percent less likely to consume the recommended fruits and vegetables than those in counties that have supermarkets.

There are larger implications from the lack of access to healthy food. Residents in areas without access to good food have poor physical and economic health, due to costs in obtaining food (transportation) and the costs associated with poor health. Local businesses suffer due to an unhealthy workforce, and state and local governments face increasing health care costs and the loss of tax revenues when residents leave a jurisdiction to purchase food. According to the University of North Carolina, rural food deserts will increase as rural populations decline, and the food industry continues to shift distribution to larger superstores in higher population areas. Just another of the many reasons we need to change this food system now. What we're doing today is just not fair. Healthy food is essential for "life, liberty, and the pursuit of happiness," and our food system is just not delivering it to all of its citizens.

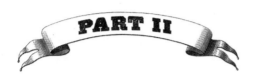

THE FIX

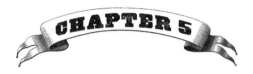

A NEW VIEW OF NUTRITION

We are now waking up to the negative effects of poor nutrition on our health. The good news is that there's a lot of information available and a new breed of food bloggers and doctors who are showing us a better way to eat—one that puts a focus on sustainably produced whole foods.

> *Let food be thy medicine, and*
> *medicine be thy food.*
>
> —HIPPOCRATES

All right. I know you may be bummed out after reading about everything that's gone wrong—though I hope you're also fired up to make some change—so now let's get into all that is going right. Because there's a lot. And let's start with one of the things that is popping up all over America: advocates for a new way of eating.

We've seen a steady rise in the number of books, movies, and websites dedicated to opening people's eyes to the ill effects of our processed foods. The demand for health coaches, a relatively new profession, has grown exponentially over the past 20 years—more than 40,000 coaches have graduated from the Institute for Integrative Nutrition alone! More of us today are relying on the expertise and education of dieticians and nutritionists, and I have worked with many of them over my career in Congress to help me understand the links between our diet and our national health. Many people I meet tell me that they have started to think for themselves about what's good and bad for them rather than just living by the government's food guidelines—and even those have undergone a makeover in the past few years (although much more work needs to be done).

Sadly, a lot of the people advocating for a better food system these days have come to their position because they've experienced a traumatic health crisis, but the work they've been doing is great because it's given a personal, real-life voice to some of the issues we're facing. They have been working to inspire change, and we can see the impact it's having in our communities, our schools, and our families.

Kris Carr, who wrote the foreword to this book, has been on the cutting edge of inspiring what she refers to as a Crazy Sexy Wellness Revolution since she was diagnosed with cancer in her early 30s. The juice and smoothie craze has taken the country by storm, and you can find juice bars and books on creating these concoctions on lists of top-selling books across America. And there are numerous "mommy blogs" that spread the word about healthy eating to mothers around the world. There's no denying that the individuals working to promote healthier eating are having an impact.

In addition to informing the powerful voices we find in popular culture, a new wave of medical doctors are looking at health in a different way, and starting to open our eyes to the effects of poor nutrition. These doctors, who refer to their practice as functional medicine, take the view that the pains, symptoms, and issues that manifest themselves can best be addressed by finding out what the root *cause* of the problems are—and often what they find is a problem with how people eat. That sounds like something most doctors would do, but in point of fact, they don't often do so. They prescribe a pill and leave it at that. Next patient, please.

When my wife, Andrea, got sick—and I mean really sick, to the point where she could hardly make it up the stairs—I experienced firsthand the power of what functional-medicine doctors have learned over years of treating people. When Andrea started experiencing symptoms, no one could figure out what was wrong with her. She was down to 90 pounds. In my eyes, my wife is the most beautiful woman in the world, but she was way too skinny. She looked unhealthy. Various doctors checked for cancer, reproductive system issues, and a host of other possible maladies. Nothing. Some kind of film would cover her eyes, and they couldn't figure that out either. The physical toll was excruciating, but the mental and emotional toll made things much worse.

Making a Difference:
Kris Carr, Crazy Sexy Wellness

In 2003, at age 31, Kris Carr was a rising star. Her agent called her "the Julia Roberts of advertising." The willowy, green-eyed blonde with an infectious smile had starred in two Bud Light commercials that ran during the Super Bowl, to great acclaim. In February, she came home to New York from the Sarasota Film Festival, where a film of hers had debuted, and decided to detox from a spate of pretty heavy partying. She had a lot to celebrate, but her life was about to change in a big way.

Instead of starting to feel better, she started feeling a lot worse. She was short of breath and had severe abdominal cramping. After a few misdiagnoses, on Valentine's Day the word came in: cancer in the lining of her blood vessels and lungs so rare that only two to three hundred cases are diagnosed yearly across the country. Stage IV. No operation. No cure.

Carr embarked on a search for healing. She found many doctors who didn't seem to care about the patient or take a holistic view, until she found Dr. George Demetri at the Dana-Farber Cancer Institute in Boston, who believed that she could do more than "watch and wait"; she could live. She evolved a philosophy of Crazy Sexy Wellness, and she defines the two key words as follows: Crazy = out-of-the-box, game-changing, trailblazing; Sexy = empowered, whole, awake, active (or activist). And she knows that how you eat is central to healthy living. Her *Crazy Sexy Diet* and *Crazy Sexy Kitchen* are *New York Times* bestsellers. Eleven years after her diagnosis, she's thriving with cancer, inspiring others to live to the fullest no matter what, and spreading the word that nutrition makes a very big difference when it comes to living well.

One day someone at Andrea's doctor's office mentioned a gluten allergy. She read like crazy and found out everything she could about gluten and celiac disease. Gluten—a protein that is found in foods processed from wheat and some other grain species—is well-known to all of us by now, since an increasing number of people have been found to be gluten intolerant, either because the condition itself is on the rise or doctors have gotten better at diagnosing it.

Dr. Hyman told us that more than 3 million Americans have celiac disease, and more than 20 million are gluten intolerant. One would imagine a little bit of gluten couldn't be that harmful; maybe it could give you the sniffles. But the reality is that gluten intolerance isn't like an allergy to pollen that makes your eyes water. It's excruciating for many people. Andrea worked hard to limit gluten in her diet. No bread, no pasta; she followed it to a T. But even trace amounts could set off a reaction, and inevitably there was always some cross-contamination. It would come out of nowhere. A salad being made in the same kitchen as the homemade pizza shell or fresh bread. Her stomach would become bloated and hard. It was a dramatic cramping pain that hurt her and everyone else who loved her. We felt helpless and on edge all the time.

Luckily, as fate would have it, I went to an event where Dr. Mark Hyman was speaking. Mark is a family physician and eight-time *New York Times* best-selling author, who was recently profiled in a *New York Times* feature that talked about his work with Bill and Hillary Clinton, not only on their personal health, but also on national health and nutrition strategy. After an evening listening to him explain his approach, I asked him about my wife. It's my very good fortune that he offered to help her.

A few months later, we made the ten-hour drive to see Mark at his practice in Lenox, Massachusetts. When we got to his office, I couldn't believe how things started. After a few niceties, he got on his computer and he started asking questions. The questions ranged from "Were you born natural or cesarean section?" to "What illnesses did you experience as a child and how were they treated?" to "What was your diet like as a kid? As a young adult? Now?" to "How is the relationship with your ex-husband?"

He went all the way back to birth and traced her medical, physical, and emotional history up to the day we were in his office. Why? Because, for doctors who are dedicated to functional medicine, all of these elements contribute to our health, or lack thereof. He does this with every patient he sees. Everyone gets special treatment. I love it. It turns out that for many people, including Andrea, the root is found deep in past behavior and experiences. All the way back to how things went on your day of birth.

Dr. Hyman's diagnosis was that years of antibiotic use, mostly as a young child, and lots of processed and fast food at a young age, destroyed the bacteria in her gut. She had wiped out most of the good bacteria in her intestines with all the antibiotics. There was also an overgrowth of bad bacteria and yeast. I won't get into all the details, but basically, he put her on a program of supplements, medications, and food that would "rebuild her gut."

After just a few weeks, we started to see the difference. She put on weight because her stomach was able to absorb the vitamins and minerals from the food she ate.

She felt a lot better. And, after several weeks, she had no cross-contamination issues. She still couldn't eat pasta or bread, but she could eat just about everything else. This was a significant turnaround in a short period of time, a miracle in my eyes.

One of the big things that this experience did for me—in addition to restoring my wife's health—is that it opened my eyes to just how powerful good, healthy, fresh, real food is. And on the other end of the spectrum, how dangerous fake foods are.

In addition to Mark's work, I have gotten to know and follow the work of Dr. James Gordon, founder and director of the Center for Mind-Body Medicine; Dr. Christiane Northrup, a pioneer in women's health, who emphasizes the unity of the physical, emotional, and spiritual aspects of our well-being; and Dr. Andrew Weil, founder and director of the Arizona Center for Integrative Medicine. I look forward to a day when physicians in every town in America have greater understanding of how connected diet and stress are to our well-being.

> "When I use the words *eating well*, I mean using food not only to influence health and well-being but to satisfy the senses, providing pleasure and comfort. In addition to supplying the basic needs of the body for calories and nutrients, an optimum diets should also reduce the risks of disease and fortify the body's defenses and intrinsic mechanisms of healing."
>
> —DR. ANDREW WEIL

These pioneering doctors, and the many thousands of their colleagues taking functional and integrative approaches to our health care, all emphasize the importance of nutrition, which frankly no doctor in my entire life had ever discussed with me in any form whatsoever! And I know I'm hardly alone in that. Sadly, one of the reasons for this is because nutrition is not a significant part of the curriculum at most medical schools.

||||||||||||||||||||||||||||||||||||||||||||||||||||||||||||||||||||||||||||||||||||||||||||||||||||||||||||||||||

MEDICAL SCHOOLS AND NUTRITION

The prestigious National Academy of Sciences commissioned a report called "Nutrition Education in U.S. Medical Schools." It was a joint effort of the Committee on Nutrition in Medical Education, the Food and Nutrition Board, the Commission on Life Sciences, and the National Research Council. It opened with these momentous words:

> As the American public becomes increasingly aware of the importance of nutrition in health maintenance and disease prevention and treatment, physicians are frequently expected to provide their patients with accurate, up-to-date information and guidance concerning diet, food, and health. This increased public demand for nutrition information, along with growing recognition of the integral role of nutrition in health, has contributed to a heightened awareness within the medical community of the need to provide physicians with adequate training in this area. The Food and Nutrition Board (FNB) of the National Research Council viewed the question of adequate and appropriate nutrition education in medical schools to be of sufficient national concern to warrant assessment.

And assess they did. They recommended that medical students in our country receive a minimum of 25 hours of nutrition instruction. The frightening thing is that this report came out in 1985, and not much has happened to remedy this situation. Here's a report from 2010, from researchers at the University of North Carolina, published in the *Journal of the American Academy of Medical Colleges*, that summarizes nicely the progress over the two decades following this initial call to action:

> Of the 105 schools answering questions about courses and contact hours, only 26 (25%) required a dedicated nutrition course; in 2004, 32 (30%) of 106 schools did. Overall, medical students received 19.6 contact hours of nutrition instruction during their medical school careers (range: 0–70 hours); the average in 2004 was 22.3 hours. Only 28 (27%) of the 105 schools met the minimum 25 required hours set by the National Academy of Sciences; in 2004, 40 (38%) of 104 schools did so.

> Conclusion: The amount of nutrition education that medical students receive continues to be inadequate.

You got that right. That's why your doctor is quicker to offer a pill than to talk about nutrition, and why the medical profession is not a major force in improving the American way of food. That's also why I drafted legislation to do something about it. The Expanding Nutrition's Role in Curricula and Healthcare Act (ENRICH Act) provides grants to medical schools if they integrate nutritional instruction into their curriculum.

‖‖

Thankfully, we have doctors who focus on nutrition to give us advice, and I believe the best way for us to reverse the current health trends is to build the new food system around their recommendations.

Here are just a few of their nutrition-related recommendations:

- Good nutrition is essential for preventing disease. It's true that diet, exercise, mind-set, and stress management all play a role in prevention, but nutrition is the most prominent element. As Dr. Weil told me, "A healthy diet is the cornerstone of a healthy lifestyle."

- We should eat a diet that does not promote inflammation in the body. Dr. Weil points out that much of our current food supply—packaged foods with artificial additives, colorings, flavors, and so on—actually causes inflammation. While this is the body's natural protective response, chronic inflammation can lead to many diseases, particularly age-related conditions.

- Avoid processed foods as much as possible. Processed foods, especially sugar, act like addictive drugs in the body, causing us to crave more and more of them even though they are detrimental to our health.

When I asked if we could put these ideas into some easy-to-follow guidelines, here are some of the main points I got:

- Cut out or cut way down on your intake of highly processed foods, avoiding synthetic chemicals, additives, coloring, and preservatives. If it's packaged in a pretty box, bag, or can, it's likely not going to be as healthy as you want it to be.

- Emphasize whole foods—high fiber and low starch—with, as Dr. Gordon says, "foods as close as possible to their natural state." As some people say, "Shop around the edge of the market."

- Limit grains and emphasize leafy vegetables and fruits. And when you're searching for what to eat, aim for a variety so you can get a greater spectrum of the nutrients, vitamins, and minerals that are essential for health.

- Limit or eliminate processed sugar. Yes, we all love cookies, but cutting down on sugar can have extreme benefits for both your health and your energy levels.

- Watch out for refined vegetable oils, including canola oil, corn oil, safflower oil, peanut oil, rapeseed oil, and soybean oil. These sneaky oils go through intensive processing, which often results in the creation of trans-fatty acids, or partially hydrogenated oils, which raise your bad cholesterol and lower your good cholesterol, increasing your risk for heart disease and stroke.

- Eat more fish. Fish are high in omega-3 fatty acids, which have been shown to reduce inflammation and play an essential role in healthy cell function. However, you shouldn't just eat *any* fish. Some have big problems with mercury contamination, so check out a list of healthy seafood available in your region at Seafood Watch (seafoodwatch.org).

- Eat meat that is raised antibiotic-free and, in the case of beef, grass-fed, which is higher in nutrients like beta-carotene and lutein, and lower in cholesterol. The more an animal lives in its natural environment, eating the food it was meant to eat, the more beneficial nutrients it will provide. Plus it's tastier and fills you up faster!

- Enjoy healthy fats like nuts and nut butters, avocados, and cold-pressed oils (olive oil, flax oil), and limit unhealthy fats, such as butter, cream, and fats from red meat.

- If you would like to enjoy alcohol, which in moderate amounts has beneficial qualities according to some research (particularly red wine), it can be a standard part of a healthy diet, but don't start drinking as a health strategy.

- And one more thing that everyone seems to agree on: enjoy your food, savor it, and eat foods that *actually taste good*, not just those that fool your senses with sugar, fat, and salt, and leave you unsatisfied a few minutes later.

- And this advice is from me: If you do cheat a little bit, enjoy it. Nothing's worse

than straying from your diet and then
feeling guilty about it. Be disciplined for
the good of your own health, but if you
sneak an occasional Dairy Queen sundae,
or breakfast roll from Panera Bread, or Five
Guys hamburger, just be sure to enjoy it.

Naturally, not every nutrition-minded doctor will agree on every single detail. And there will be some wacky outliers of course who recommend a diet they discovered in a flash of brilliance while hiking in the high Andes, but diet fads are just that: fads.

But this is good; we shouldn't expect total agreement. Groups of humans don't do that. I should know; I'm in Congress. But, I think we can find a kind of consensus diet, and we need a system that supports that, including reimbursing doctors for taking the time to teach and train patients to improve lifestyle in order to achieve improved health outcomes.

One aspect of that is to refine the food recommendations that our government uses. While Michelle Obama did improve it from its previous state, for which she deserves a lot of credit, creating My Plate (choosemyplate .gov) in place of the old food pyramid, it still needs work. While it does recommend that half of your plate should be filled with fruits and vegetables, it still leaves a quarter of your plate for grains—specifying that at least half should be whole grains—which means that half of those can be refined grains. Luckily, there are many alternative food recommendations out there. Dr. Weil's food pyramid (shown on the following page) is one example that helps illustrate some of the concepts I learned as I talked to these functional-medicine doctors.

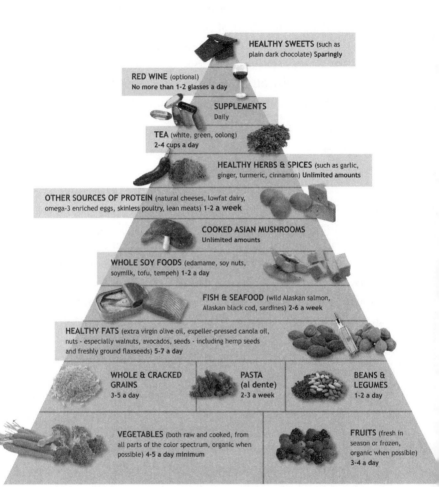

HEALTHY SWEETS (such as plain dark chocolate) **Sparingly**

RED WINE (optional)
No more than 1-2 glasses a day

SUPPLEMENTS
Daily

TEA (white, green, oolong)
2-4 cups a day

HEALTHY HERBS & SPICES (such as garlic, ginger, turmeric, cinnamon) **Unlimited amounts**

OTHER SOURCES OF PROTEIN (natural cheeses, lowfat dairy, omega-3 enriched eggs, skinless poultry, lean meats) **1-2 a week**

COOKED ASIAN MUSHROOMS
Unlimited amounts

WHOLE SOY FOODS (edamame, soy nuts, soymilk, tofu, tempeh) **1-2 a day**

FISH & SEAFOOD (wild Alaskan salmon, Alaskan black cod, sardines) **2-6 a week**

HEALTHY FATS (extra virgin olive oil, expeller-pressed canola oil, nuts - especially walnuts, avocados, seeds - including hemp seeds and freshly ground flaxseeds **5-7 a day**

WHOLE & CRACKED GRAINS
3-5 a day

PASTA
(al dente)
2-3 a week

BEANS & LEGUMES
1-2 a day

VEGETABLES (both raw and cooked, from all parts of the color spectrum, organic when possible) **4-5 a day minimum**

FRUITS (fresh in season or frozen, organic when possible) **3-4 a day**

Courtesy of www.DrWeil.com

As healthier options become more accessible, people can create their own diet from what's available to them, whether it's the kind of diet recommended by the doctors I've mentioned here, or vegan, vegetarian, paleo, no-wheat, and so on. The common factor is that the food available to them in the marketplace is healthy at affordable prices, which is bound to lead to a higher level of health and well-being in the country. Hey, nobody used to wear seat belts. Now, almost everyone does. Same with teeth brushing. Now, not brushing your teeth is definitely considered a bad idea.

I know that Americans are not suddenly going to take all these recommendations, but there's no point in gorging on supersized french fries and a 24-ounce soda while debating the fine differences between the many different doctor-recommended diets. The consensus seems clear: *more whole foods and less processed food will increase health and save lives.*

■ ■ ■

WHAT YOU CAN DO

While reading a nutrition label is not an easy thing to do, make it a goal to learn what each of the lines means for your health. Check out this website to get some of the guidelines: www.fda.gov/food/ingredientspackaging labeling/labelingnutrition/ucm274593.htm.

Good nutrition starts right at home. Take a look in your cupboards, fridge, and freezer. If you've now become an expert in label reading, this step will be a snap, but even if you didn't you'll be able to improve your food supply. Really read the ingredients on the foods you most commonly buy. If you want to make a dramatic shift, throw out anything that has fake, unpronounceable ingredients in it. If you're looking for more gradual change, find a couple of processed foods that you can do without. Make it a goal to replace those things with fresh, healthy, whole foods. Remember, you vote with your dollars at the supermarket.

In a journal—or even a document on your computer—keep track of everything you eat over the course of a normal week and how you feel following the consumption of those foods. Can you identify anything that made you feel low-energy? Did you experience a high and then a crash? Did eating something full of sugar inspire other cravings in you? Simple awareness will help you make better food choices.

Eating fresh means eating what's in season in the region where you are. The Natural Resources Defense Council has put together a website where you can click on any U.S. state to see what's in season during any month of the year: www.simplesteps.org/eat-local.

You may have heard of Meatless Monday, a program that was started in 2003 in association with the Johns Hopkins Bloomberg School of Public Health. Their goal is to influence people—and even entire communities—to embrace the idea of going meat-free for one day each week. As their website says, "Skipping meat one day a week is good for you, great for your nation's health, and fantastic for the planet." This movement has now spread to 34 countries across the world.

Meatlessmonday.com has great resources and recipes to help you implement this idea in your own life. And if you're really inspired, they have toolkits to help spread the word through your community.

The makers of the movie *Fed Up*, released in May 2014, want viewers to take action, so they have set up a challenge to help people cut sugar out of their diets for ten days. See www.fedupmovie.com to sign up for the challenge and to download a toolkit to help educate others about food issues in America.

Great things happen in small groups. With any of these approaches, you can put together a small band of brothers and sisters to get things started. Whether it's Meatless Mondays or the Fed Up Challenge, we need a support system to not only get us started, but to sustain us so we can benefit personally and raise awareness throughout our community. It's the same for the community projects. Build a small team and watch success come your way.

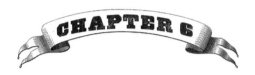

POLICY ADVOCACY

A new, vibrant, and exciting vision of our food system has been emerging over the past few decades, and yet the entrenched powers that run the current food system are increasing their hold on the status quo. If we want to see a new way of food, we need to campaign for it, focusing on a few key areas where we need change now.

> *As soon as one legislator loses their job over the way they vote on food issues, it will send a clear message to Congress: We are organized. We're strong. Yes, we have a food movement, and it's coming for you.*
>
> —Tom Colicchio

Now, let's jump from the personal level to the national and local level—information about what's happening to reform our broken food policy. When we have to reform a system, we usually find that there is a clash of wills. And that's what's going on with food: The wills of the moms and dads of America who desire to feed their children healthy food are pitted against the will, and money, of the food industrial complex—the agriculture industry giants and food processors who have a vise grip on the current system and want to keep it just like it is. It benefits them, but it doesn't benefit us anywhere near how much it should.

In the United States these battles come to a head in legislatures in our state capitals and in Washington, DC. These are places where conflict comes to happen. As a congressman, I actually relish these situations because this is how great change can take place. The bigger the issue, the more I want to be in the middle of it. It's like the old Irish saying, "Is this a private fight or can anyone get in?" I'm waist-deep in the food issue now and the big moneyed interests are out in full force—with armies of lawyers—putting millions of dollars into our political system to prevent parents from knowing exactly what is in their children's food and to maintain the capability to keep farmers dependent on their products.

The vision of an American food system that a few massive companies have promoted needs to be challenged by citizens who care more about the health of our people than the wealth of our corporations. As I've been saying, a new and vibrant vision of food in America has been developing for decades, and it's reaching a tipping point. I believe once such a new vision is presented more widely, people will gravitate toward it. And they will support it with their advocacy and their votes—both in the marketplace and the ballot box.

Happily there are a few intrepid groups working to make change right now. I've spent a lot of time getting to know them, and from their counsel, I've gleaned what seem to me to be the five campaigns we need to work on: GMO labeling, breaking the seed monopoly, rebalancing farm bill subsidies, making crop insurance more equitable, and reducing antibiotic use. Let's dive deeper into these issues.

Campaign #1: Require GMO Labeling

John Mackey, CEO of Whole Foods, has said, "Democratic capitalism remains by far the best way to organize society to create prosperity, growth, freedom, self-actualization, and even equality." I agree. The free enterprise system can be a powerful force for good—when it's allowed to operate properly and freely.

> "Democratic capitalism remains by far the best way to organize society to create prosperity, growth, freedom, self-actualization, and even equality."
>
> —John Mackey

And the most efficient way to let the market work freely is to provide the customer with the most information possible. Laws have evolved to protect consumers from getting scammed or hurt by certain products. In a much crueler world the approach was "caveat emptor," let the buyer beware. Fortunately, the buyer gets a little help these days to even the playing field.

We get appraisals and inspections before we purchase a home or car. If we are misled when we purchase a car, we are protected by lemon laws. If someone tries to manipulate an odometer by making a car seem like it has less mileage than it actually has, it's a criminal offense. If we are to take out a loan for a home, especially now after the financial crisis, we must read and sign numerous documents that spell out all of the detailed information about the terms of the agreement. These laws and processes are meant to increase the amount of information a consumer has on which to make a decision. I think most Americans would agree that hiding information about a product is unethical and unfair. If we have all the information and make a decision that doesn't work out, it's no one's fault but our own. And we all have examples of making those bad decisions. But, what is mind-boggling is that the food industry wants to hide what's in the food they grow, manufacture, and deliver to our local grocery store or, worse yet, to our schools. Sorry, but we want to know, and there is a movement building to knock down these walls of secrecy and let in the sunshine. If we

> "The government subsidizes corn, wheat and soy, but there's no reason that unhealthy processed foods should cost less than a peach. It's a choice we make— a bad choice."
>
> —TOM COLICCHIO

expect full disclosure about a car or house we're thinking of buying, why not the food we eat?

You may be familiar with Tom Colicchio, the head judge on Bravo's hit television show *Top Chef.* He isn't only a top-flight chef and businessperson, he is also a passionate advocate for reforms in our food system. He sits on the board of directors for Food Policy Action, a progressive organization that holds politicians accountable by monitoring their votes on food issues and sharing that information with the general public. Their work makes a vital contribution to Americans who are interested in changing the food system, by letting us know which public officials need to be persuaded to change their positions or be voted out of office. I really appreciate when a very busy guy like Tom gets engaged in the political process.

In the span of just a couple weeks I received a mass e-mail from Tom, and had meetings with representatives from Stonyfield Farm, the world's leading organic yogurt producer; Ben & Jerry's, the famous ice cream company; and three progressive organizations promoting major changes to our food system: Food Policy Action, Environmental Working Group (EWG), and The National Farmers Union. In each case, the top priority these people were advocating for was the same: transparency on what is in our food.

The representative from Ben & Jerry's, Christopher Miller, whose title is social mission activism manager, told me that his company is committed to having all its products GMO labeled by the end of 2014 and is a partner in Just Label It, a national coalition of groups calling on the FDA to require labeling. He also emphasized that the United States is behind in its approach to GMOs compared to Europe. "We sell into twenty-four other countries around the world. A number of the countries we export to have mandatory GMO labeling. That makes it complicated for us. If we want to export from Vermont to the European Union, for example, we have to have production in Europe in order to effectively meet the EU standards for what qualifies as non-GMO. In a perfect world, there would be a uniform GMO labeling framework consistent with the framework in other countries, then we could export product that was produced here in Vermont and have it pass regulatory scrutiny in the EU." In other words, our country is falling behind and some of our most innovative producers, who support sustainable, healthy agriculture, are paying for it.

Wood Turner is the vice president of sustainability innovation at Stonyfield Organic, which produces all-organic dairy products and distributes across the country. He explained to me that they deal with small farms (around 80 cows) and cooperatives made up of small farms, and many of these are family farms that have been having a tough time. The farmers' toughest problem is getting organic, non-GMO feed. If the market grows for non-GMO food, then the market will grow for non-GMO feed, making these operations more viable. A key part of Stonyfield's philosophy is to support small operations and complete transparency to the consumer of the supply chain that is bringing food to their table.

Apparently, not everyone likes transparency quite so much. Legislation introduced by Rep. Mike Pompeo from Kansas would block any federal or state action to require labeling of foods made with genetically engineered in-

> "More than 90 percent of Americans support labeling of GE foods."
>
> —SCOTT FABER

gredients. Yes, in 2014 there is legislation being presented to hide information from the public. And we wonder why Congress's approval rating is so low.

"More than 90 percent of Americans support labeling of GE foods," Scott Faber, of the EWG, told me. "It's clear the public wants to know what's in their food, but if Representative Pompeo has his way, no one will have that right." In 2013, according to the United States Department of Agriculture, 90 percent of corn planted in the U.S. was genetically modified. We need a label to tell us what is and what isn't. We don't need a big government program here; we just need a label. Let the consumer know. Is that too much to ask?

Consumers *must* know which foods are GE and which are not. Parents and other consumers will choose to avoid foods containing poison, spurring the growth of markets for non-GMO foods. As demand for non-GE food increases, more farmers will start planting them. The increase in supply will keep costs in check.

CAMPAIGN #2: BREAK THE MONOPOLY, PARTICULARLY ON SEED, WHICH IS ANTI-FARMER AND ANTI-COMPETITIVE

The American farmer has always represented the tenacity, resiliency, and freedom provided by the American way of life. They work long hours, work the land, and bring their values of community and compassion to the American fabric. That is why it is sad to see them getting stuck under the thumb of a few monopolistic corporations. Ken Roseboro, the editor and publisher of *The Organic & Non-GMO Report*, in an article titled "The GMO Seed Monopoly: Fewer Choices, Higher Prices," wrote:

> Economists say that when four companies control 40 percent of a market, it's no longer competitive. That's apparently the situation now with U.S. corn and soybean seed markets. According to AgWeb [an agricultural news website], the "big four" biotech seed companies—Monsanto,

Making a Difference: Dan Barber, Political Chef

Many chefs today want to get out of the kitchen and do something about the food system, and they're helping to lead the charge in the real food revolution. Dan Barber is a leader in this new breed, and he aims to change the American way of food. A smart, New York City kid, Barber seemed destined to earn a living from his brain. After getting a degree in political science and English from Tufts in Boston, he decided he wanted to become a chef. His dad told him, "Son, I love books, but I don't read for a living."

But Barber has indeed brought his brains and his political education into his work. He has a restaurant located within the Stone Barns Center for Food and Agriculture on the former Rockefeller estate in the lovely lower Hudson River valley in upstate New York. Its mission: increase awareness of healthy, seasonal, and sustainable food; train farmers in resilient, restorative farming techniques; and educate children about the sources of their food, and prepare them to steward the land that provides it.

Barber is a regular Op-Ed columnist in *The New York Times*; serves on the President's Council on Physical Fitness, Sports, and Nutrition; and is also a member of the Advisory Board to the Harvard Medical School Center for Health and the Global Environment. His 2014 book, *The Third Plate: Field Notes on the Future of Food*, asks us to vote with our forks and knives. He advocates that we buy at farmers' markets, grow some food ourselves, cook, talk to the grocery store manager about what we want to see, and vote with food policy as a central concern.

DuPont/Pioneer, Syngenta, and Dow AgroSciences—own 80 percent of the U.S. corn market and 70 percent of the soybean business. They also control more than half the world's seed supply.

Our farmers are on the other side of this rigged game. Genetically engineered seeds have increased in price by 230 percent from 2000 to 2010. The average cost per acre for soy has increased by 325 percent, and corn by 259 percent. Non-GE corn varieties have been reduced by 67 percent while GE varieties have increased by 6.7 percent from 2005 to 2010. Farmers face an increase in costs and a decrease in options. If it looks like a monopoly and smells like manure, you know it stinks for our farmers.

Large food producers are just as exploitive, with behemoths like Archer Daniels Midland and Cargill running the show. Cargill is the largest privately owned company in America. These big businesses are vertically integrated, so they are in control of everything from the seeds to grains, the fertilizers to pesticides, and, sometimes, even the processing of the food until it lands at your supermarket. As A. V. Krebs, research director at Prairie Fire Rural Action in Iowa, has written:

> Cargill and Continental Grain together control 50 percent of all grain exported from the United States. Cargill has also become the second-largest meat packer in the country. Cargill, Iowa Beef Processors, and ConAgra together slaughter close to 80 percent of all the meat

slaughtered in the United States. Four companies—General Foods, General Mills, Kellogg's and Quaker Oats—dominate almost 90 percent of an ever-growing cold cereal market. When four companies control 40 percent or more of the market, economists usually consider the market to be oligopolistic.

This campaign is a tough uphill slog, make no mistake about it, because the companies controlling seed are so powerful, but as Michael Pollan emphasized to me, to remove this kind of independence, in the form of control over their own seed, is unfair and un-American, no matter what your politics are. While crisscrossing the country giving talks, he has found that farmers are widely supportive of freeing the seed monopoly. They believe in independence. One of the groups working on this campaign is the Open Source Seed Initiative, a group of scientists, citizens, plant breeders, farmers, seed companies, and gardeners, whose motto is "Free the Seed." Breaking the seed monopoly is also one of the key campaigns of the grassroots food advocacy group Food Democracy Now!

Campaign #3: Rebalance the Farm Bill Toward Small and Medium-Sized Farmers

I know many Americans, myself included, are concerned about our country's long-term fiscal health. And many taxpayers are feeling squeezed and have trouble making ends meet for their families. If we reform our agriculture system, we can reduce government spending—remember that $292 billion in taxes?—but we can do something else as well. We can improve our own health and the health of the planet.

Sadly, your local, sustainable farmer from whom you buy your grass-fed beef or your fresh fruits and vegetables is not getting much of our tax money. Neither is the urban farm that is operating in the city you live in, turning blighted communities into havens of fresh, healthy food. The money isn't going to help schools set up classrooms to teach our children about horticulture and nutrition at a young age. It's not going to the vast majority of farmers. This money is going to a small handful of farms that grow crops for the food industrial complex.

Of the $292 billion spent on subsidies over the past 18 years, 75 percent went to only 10 percent of the farms and businesses. You can see why the large corporate agricultural interests have spent so much on political campaigns.

How are the hardworking small and medium-sized farmers doing (the ones we think of when we see a big red barn a few miles outside of our town)? Well, the bottom 80 percent of farmers from 1995 to 2012 received on average—get ready for it—$604 a year! A lobbyist can spend that on dinner in one night. In some states half of the farmers didn't get a dime. Small family farmers have seen increased prices for seed and less choice, and they get a pittance from the government while the top 1 percent of the farmers run off with the spoils. This upper echelon of farmers use their subsidy money to buy seed supplied by the biotech seed companies, who are also benefiting quite well from the current system.

Thank goodness there are active groups working toward this aim with their own lobbyists. The Environmental Working Group, the National Sustainable

Agriculture Coalition, the National Farmers Union, and a number of other organizations are getting representatives to Capitol Hill to present the other side of the argument. If you want to get involved in the campaign to rebalance the subsidies we're giving to farmers, these are the people to pay attention to and get behind.

I agree with them that it makes more sense to put some of our tax money into the smaller farmers and allow them to have more stability and security, while also providing fresh, healthy food that is affordable for all of our citizens. At the very least, we should turn off the government spigot and let the free market work, so the price of the bad food will rise to a level that reflects its true price. This will create a much more competitive market for the vast majority of farmers and growers.

As we transition to a new system, we also need to ensure small and midsize farmers' operations can be profitable and stay in business. They're the lifeblood of the new food system, and we need to help them. Many of them have invested a lot of money and mortgaged their homes and businesses to try to succeed in a very risky business environment. While I prefer not to directly subsidize businesses, I believe these farmers are an important exception. They have razor-thin profit margins, and any kind of international volatility, unscrupulous global commodity trading, or natural disaster can throw crops and prices into a tailspin. That is a dangerous situation when we are talking about our nation's food supply. Some intervention and insurance is needed to make sure we have a steady supply of food. Investing in smaller, healthier, more sustainable farming operations is a good investment of our tax dollars. Propping up the current system is not.

Campaign #4: End the Scams in the New Farm Bill

Mike Lavender is a tall and bearded fellow with a quiet and straightforward demeanor. He was dressed in a suit and tie the day I met him, but he gave off a very laid-back vibe, despite what he knows about how much needs to be reformed in our food system. I met him in my Washington office as I was trying to better and more fully understand our country's agriculture policies. He is the agriculture reform coordinator for the Environmental Working Group. They are leading the charge when it comes to organizing and arming us with information to bring change to our food policies.

Mike explained to me that the new farm bill has moved from direct payments to farmers to crop insurance. On the surface, it sounds like a good reform: instead of directly subsidizing farmers no matter what the conditions, you pay them to have insurance they can draw on if things go bad. But when you look at how it really works, the story is not so neat or pretty.

> "It's farmers and taxpayers—two groups Congress claims to care about—who are hurt the most by wasteful and misdirected farm subsidies. At a time of record farm profits and record federal deficits, farmers have been the first to admit that these programs need to change."
>
> —Mike Lavender

For starters, only about a dozen companies in the U.S. provide crop insurance. In the new farm bill they get to split close to $1.3 billion for "overhead expenses." In addition to the overhead payments to the insurance companies, the premiums paid by the farmers are subsidized, at an average of 60 percent of the cost. The premiums for cotton are subsidized to the tune of 80 percent. These payments, as usual, are going to the top farmers, not small and medium-sized farmers. And there is no limit on premium support. As a result, according to research by the Environmental Working Group, 26 policyholders received more than $1 million apiece in taxpayer-funded crop insurance subsidies in 2011, and more than 10,000 policyholders received more than $100,000 each.

According to Craig Cox, EWG's senior vice president for agriculture and natural resources, the 2014 farm bill that I voted against failed to "fix the flawed crop insurance program by putting some limit on the amount of subsidies that farm operations can get to lower the cost of their insurance policies. The largest and most financially secure farm businesses harvest most of those subsidies."

Let me be clear: crop insurance is an important and essential component of our nation's agriculture policy. Many farmers in my district are still farmers today because crop insurance helped them weather difficult times. Most of those farmers paid their full premium themselves, as opposed to having their payment subsidized. Crop insurance must be available and accessible to our farmers in their times of greatest need. It must be there to support the small, medium, and specialty crop farmers. So, my issue isn't with crop insurance, it is with how the current system needs to be right-sized and refocused.

Another part of the recently enacted farm bill is the Price Loss Coverage program. Here's how it works, as described by the Environmental Working Group:

> The program puts price floors under commodity crops—and sets them in stone. These "floors" are really high because they're based on the record-breaking crop prices of recent years. When Congress was writing these so-called "reference prices" into law, the projections were exceedingly optimistic. Even so, the Congressional Budget Office forecasted that the Price Loss Coverage program would end up costing taxpayers $13.1 billion over the next 10 years.

Now, according to a report issued by the Food and Agricultural Policy Research Institute, it's going to cost at least $21 billion more than projected. The Institute's analysis shows that the Price Loss Coverage program will now likely cost taxpayers upwards of $34.2 billion over the next ten years. That's because the latest projections of crop prices by the USDA predict that prices for corn, soybeans, wheat, and other crops not only are not going to climb in coming years, they may likely drop below the floors in the new bill, and stay there, triggering the massive payments mentioned above. One of the promises of the new farm bill was that it would provide *budget savings*. That promise is looking pretty thin at this point.

|||||||||||||||||||||||||||||||||||||||||||||||||||||||||||||||||||||||||||||||||||||||||||||||||||||||||||||||||||||||||||||||

LEGISLATORS TO WATCH

After being in Congress for 12 years now, I've learned who the go-to leaders are in certain issue areas. Luckily, in the food, farming, and health area, there are some great people on the cutting edge of transforming the way we look at these issues.

- Sherrod Brown, senator from Ohio, is leading the charge on issues from urban agriculture to health and wellness by sponsoring or cosponsoring key pieces of legislation. He sees how these systems are all tied together and advocates forcefully that these issues are about fairness and justice for all.

- Cory Booker, senator from New Jersey, is one of the newer members of the Senate. He hosted the premiere for the documentary *Fed Up* on Capitol Hill, and is a strong advocate for a healthier food system. As former mayor of Newark, NJ, he knows how federal policies can either help or hurt citizens in their own neighborhoods.

- Rosa DeLauro, representative from Connecticut, is the most powerful voice for the health of our children. As a longtime member of the House Appropriations Committee, she advocates for a more robust Food and Drug Administration so our children are protected from the hard edges of a global economy. She is also a major force in trying to improve nutrition in our schools.

- Chellie Pingree, representative from Maine, is an organic farmer by trade and has been honored by the Environmental Working Group for her work on changing the farm bill. She is a passionate advocate for shifting the current monoculture farming system to one that favors the regional and organic farmer. Her legislation is always well researched, and because of her background she knows exactly where the system needs to go.

- Marcia Fudge, representative from Cleveland, is chair of the Congressional Black Caucus and a fierce advocate for urban agriculture. She understands the importance of reconnecting urban America to our food system and getting healthy food into our inner cities. Her legislation—the Let's Grow Act—should be a cornerstone of the new food system.

- Ron Kind, representative from Wisconsin (and a former Harvard quarterback), is a leader on reforming our farm subsidy and crop insurance program. He has been pushing reform for his entire career even when he was a lonely voice in the wilderness. His persistence has taught me a lot, and I follow his lead on many of these issues.

- Lastly, Marcy Kaptur, representative from Toledo, Ohio, understands better than anyone how powerful agriculture can be. She is the top Democrat on the Energy Appropriations Subcommittee and pushes every day for new and emerging technologies that can help with sustainability and conservation for regional and sustainable agriculture. She knows the power of urban farming and how it can tie into a broader agenda dealing with our overall energy consumption.

Campaign #5: Reduce Antibiotic and Hormone Use

Another issue that must be addressed is the heavy use of antibiotics on our farms. We're not talking about the situation where a cow gets sick and needs to go on a course of antibiotics until they are well again. That would represent occasional use. What we see in our industrialized agricultural methodology is systematic continuous use.

According to a fact sheet from the Pew Charitable Trusts, in 2011 there were 30 million pounds of antibiotics sold for use in food animal production and 8 million sold to treat sick people. That's almost four times as many antibiotics going to food animals. Why, in God's name, would we give so many antibiotics to farm animals? Here's why: cows are ruminants—mammals who are able to acquire nutrients from plant-based food by fermenting it in a specialized stomach prior to digestion. Cows evolved to have a chamber, called the rumen, that allows them to digest grass. I'll spare you all the unpleasant details of this process, but suffice it to say that it causes them to convert the grass into some pretty healthy proteins. A normal cow eating grass takes several years of grazing to get big enough to go to market. Some people who raise grass-fed cattle say three or four years is ideal.

But as we've already discussed, three or four years is too long for the current big cattle businesses. In order to speed up the process—to get the cows bigger and fattened up more quickly—the cattle industry started feeding them corn. Corn is a grain; it's high in sugar, starch, and the bad-for-you polyunsaturated fats. The problem is that the grass-loving rumen gets really out of whack when cows eat corn. And the cows get sick.

Genetically modified corn, which is grown using petroleum-based pesticides and herbicides, changes the pH levels in the belly. Sometimes this can create ulcers in the rumen, which leads to a lot of bacteria that can get into the bloodstream. The liver gets infected, too, and this could cause liver abscesses.

In order to address the sickness, cattle raisers give them—hold the applause—antibiotics. Low levels of antibiotics are actually mixed in with the corn they eat. This is a regular part of the daily diet for most cows because the current system is making them sick. On top of that they are hanging out in their own feces for extended periods of time, especially toward the end of their lives. They need antibiotics for that, too.

This heavy antibiotic use has made these miracle drugs less effective when we really need them, to fight disease, not just to make more money from beef. A September 2013 report from Consumer Reports outlined the threat that all of these antibiotics pose to our health—because we're taking so many antibiotics to combat illness and consuming so many through our food, strains of superbugs are actually developing a resistance to more and more of our antibiotics. Over two million people have gotten sick because of this problem and 23,000 people have died."If we're not careful, we will soon be in a post-antibiotic era," said Thomas Frieden, director of the U.S. Centers for Disease Control and Prevention, in September when the CDC released their report detailing drug-resistance threats. "For some patients and some microbes, we are already there." More people are dying from these staph bacteria in America than are dying of AIDS.

Once again, the Environmental Working Group is the team leading the charge on this campaign. It produces the *Meat Eater's Guide to Climate Change + Health*, which you can access on their website, where you can also learn more about how to read labels to understand when you're getting meat with fewer antibiotics, hormones, and toxins. In this case, we can vote with our dollars and our stomachs by demanding meat without these substances.

THE GOOD STUFF

An honest assessment of the most recent farm bill shows some steps in the right direction. We need to acknowledge this and use the momentum from it to make future improvements. Subsidies were eliminated for farmers who didn't experience an actual loss. There were increases in what farmers have to do with regard to conservation and incentives to encourage them to do it. Beginning farmer programs saw increased investment to help them get started by plugging them in to USDA programs like loans and help with insurance. Specialty crops saw a boost as well, and this recognition gives us something to build on.

Legislating is a tough business. I want to mention several tenacious lawmakers who slugged it out to make some of these changes. Senator Debbie Stabenow from Michigan fought extremely hard to make sure specialty crop block grants and value-added producer grants saw increased investment. She was a rock star throughout the entire farm bill process. Tim Walz, my colleague from Minnesota, was relentless and got a win by cutting subsidies to farmers who plowed native prairie to plant crops. This is a solid reform that will save the taxpayers money. Senators Durbin, Grassley, and Tim Johnson worked hard to try to get a sliding scale for crop insurance premiums to lower support for wealthy farmers. It was a strong bipartisan effort that didn't quite make it into the law, but they should be commended for their efforts. Lastly, a group of farm and conservation groups like the National Farm Bureau and National Wildlife Federation were responsible for those conservation advances I mentioned above. We must acknowledge the great work of these lawmakers and groups who have been working in the legislative trenches to enact policies that are better for both us and our farmers.

I know most of us would rather ignore what's happening in Washington, since there is so much to do day-to-day with our kids and community. But it's so important to use your voice to influence the process to make things better for your kids and community. And it is even more important to set the example for your children because these changes will not be implemented overnight. We must teach our children, so they may teach our grandchildren, and we can bend this system in the direction of health and wellness for all of us.

■ ■ ■

WHAT YOU CAN DO

The best thing you can do to move policy is to get organized and get a group of like-minded people working together on a local level.

In Ohio we have benefitted from food policy councils that bring local interest groups together in communities to help problem-solve challenges we may have with the food system. There are hundreds of these across the country. See if one of these exists in your area. If not, start a council in your local community. The Drake University Agricultural Law Center in Des Moines, Iowa, maintains an interactive map of food policy councils across the nation. You can access it at maps.google.com/maps/ms?m sid=213555848782270380380.0004729d8ff3817adc166& msa=0&dg=feature.

On a very local level, you can hold a house party to raise awareness or start a foodie group at your church, library, community group, or yoga center. If you don't have a place to meet, ask your local grocery store. They often have community meeting spaces that they will make available for free. Then, get educated on the issues. The Environmental Working Group (www.ewg .org/key-issues or www.ewg.org/take-action) and Food Policy Action (www.foodpolicyaction.org/whyitmatters .php) have great resources on their websites to help you bone up on the issues being raised in Congress. Once you feel comfortable, call your local congressperson and set up a meeting for your group. Do NOT take no for an answer. All you need is 15 to 20 minutes to explain your views. Outline the exact pieces of legislation you want them to cosponsor and vote for. Bring the whole group, the more the merrier. Trust me, your representative will pay attention if you have a good number of voters supporting your position as well. If your member responds well, write a letter saying thank you.

To demonstrate to your representative that you have real support for your position, carry out a petition drive within your local food movement, and bring the petition to Washington (or to state or local government, if that's appropriate to what you're trying to get done). The University of Kansas has an excellent online resource on community organizing called "Community Tool Box." The section on petition drives is found here: www.ctb .ku.edu/en/table-of-contents/advocacy/direct-action /petition-drive/main.

If you can't go in person, start a local letter-writing campaign to your member of Congress and the local newspapers. Politicians pay attention to which way the wind is blowing. If you can show them that public momentum is building toward supporting these new approaches, they will listen. Members of Congress always ask their staffs what people are writing in about. Make them notice you! Be a pain in the butt! Start a Facebook page and organize online. Build coalitions with other like-minded groups. Set up a booth at the local farmers' market to get signatures and e-mail lists.

I know this seems obvious, but one of the biggest powers we have in a democracy is our vote. The organization Food Policy Action promotes positive agriculture and food policies. Its team does the heavy lifting of analyzing legislation to determine which pieces of legislation will have a significant impact on our nation's food policy, and monitors every vote cast on food issues. It then grades each politician as to how often they support progressive food legislation or oppose legislation that will have a negative impact. The group's website lists these pieces of legislation along with the scores of the legislators. The higher the score, the more often they vote in ways that will help improve the food system. So go to the Food Policy Action Group's Scorecard (www .foodpolicyaction.org/FPA2013Scorecard.pdf) and look at how your elected officials vote . . . and then speak to them with *your* vote.

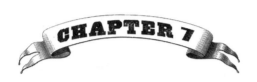

THE FARM-TO-TABLE
MOVEMENT

We need to listen to the regional farmers. We need to celebrate their work. We need to support them. They supply the kind of food we need to be eating.

Eating is an agricultural act.

—WENDELL BERRY

It was a cold day in what had been a long, snowy winter in Ohio, not the sort of day that I'm eager to spend walking around in fields. But, I had heard so many great things about Melissa and Aaron Miller's farm that I just had to meet them. Miller's Farm is just about 25 minutes from our home in Ohio and 70 miles south of Cleveland. About

15 years ago, after owning a hardware store for almost two decades, the couple decided to follow their passion and start farming. "Starting the farm was probably the difference between living and dying," Aaron said.

They started with 50 Holstein heifers and 2 beef cows. And now they run a very successful livestock business where, Melissa says, they "turn over 70 head of livestock a year, 90 pigs, 500 chickens, 100 lambs, 150 turkeys, lots of eggs, and 150 buckets of maple syrup." And if you've never had fresh maple syrup from Northeast Ohio, you don't know what you are missing!

This is a great American story in and of itself. It's great to see people who take calculated risks and then have success. But what I really love about them is that their farm is sustainable. They raise grass-fed beef and lamb and pastured pork, chickens, and turkeys. Their hens lay eggs, not in cages, but on 168 acres of land. They follow a careful plan of rotating which animals are on which pasture over a 28-day cycle. Melissa explained to me how their grass-feeding regimen works:

> We do what's called "managed intensive ro-
> tational grazing." We have big, long fields that
> have a special mixture of grass, and then we use
> a system that puts the herd into a paddock as big
> as a football field. After about 28 days, we rotate
> them out to a fresh field. This gives them the
> ideal mix of energy and routine, moving them
> all the time, so that they're not coming back
> into a place where manure has been, that way
> we don't have to use antibiotics.

The Millers have worked hard to get certified by the Food Alliance, an independent organization that has some of the highest standards for assessing sustainability. They evaluate farms on a number of practices, including safe and fair working conditions, humane treatment of animals, and stewardship of the local ecosystem. Miller's Farm passes with flying colors.

While Northeast Ohio is a tough food market, where margins are tight, the Millers are helping to grow and shape this market. Their big customer is Bon Appétit at the world-renowned Case Western Reserve University in Cleveland. In some years, Case Western has purchased up to half of their hogs. Local Food Cleveland has identified them as Superstar Farmers. They sell directly to a local restaurant in Cleveland called Fire Food & Drink as well as others in the region. They hit the farmers' markets every week.

One Saturday my wife sent me out to pick up some meat for the weekend and wouldn't you know, I bumped into Melissa and Aaron at Catullo Prime Meats, a family-run butcher shop in Youngstown. The Millers were there cooking up their meats right in the store with Danny Catullo, the third-generation butcher who has grown the business from a small-town shop to a bustling butcher shop that is a national beef distributor. Danny is always on the cutting edge (no pun intended), and now he is including Miller's meat in his portfolio. Needless to say I bought some of their amazing breakfast sausage.

The Millers work long hours and rarely take vacations, but they are able to make a decent living and send their kids to college. They just love what they do, and you can feel that love when you speak to them. And they're making a huge contribution to our local community.

They have maintained a level of independence from a system they believe has become corrupted. They aren't getting any subsidies and they're not beholden to enormous agricultural companies who control what seed you can use. They're the American farmers you think of in a Norman Rockwell painting. When I asked Melissa what she knew about the commodity farmer and the subsidies they got, she responded, "Do I know those big guys? I certainly do. Do I know that sort of business? No. We're in the food business, and food doesn't get any sort of subsidy."

I believe too many people in America are blaming our average everyday farmers for the problems caused by our food system. I don't like this. The fact of the matter is that these down-to-earth, humble farmers have been caught in the middle of a very difficult and unfair system, as I've noted. I've represented Ohio farmers in public office for the better part of 14 years. They have been an amazingly progressive force—and not just on farm issues. For people to label them as the problem does a disservice to their commitment to creating a better life for all of us. I've watched my friends in Ohio agriculture work to create and maintain a rural safety net—including everything from access to affordable health care to quality education to reliable clean energy.

I witnessed the Ohio Farm Bureau standing up for clean and renewable energy initiatives even when they were under attack by our governor and general assembly. These groups stood up for a robust transportation policy and sound funding for our schools—including a strong science, technology, engineering, and math curriculum—in addition to farm-to-school food programs.

When there was a push from outside interests to change the way Ohio agriculture houses animals, Ohio agriculture stepped up and took the lead. This was no small feat, but they did what was right for Ohio agriculture and for animal welfare. The real food revolution needs the leadership and experience of the American agricultural community. They are our allies in this effort. They are smart, open-minded, and reasonable in their approach. They are concerned about the health of their children, and they want them to live just as long or longer than themselves—to carry on the legacy. They're worried about the quality of the soil and the conservation of our land. While we have had our differences on some policy matters, I trust and respect this community like no other that I've worked with in my tenure in Congress. While I can't say if every state's agricultural groups are as enlightened as the ones in Ohio, many are open to new ideas and approaches.

In every state in our country, we need to meet the agricultural community halfway. Many farmers are stewards of family farms that are generations old. So, it is altogether appropriate for them to hesitate at literally risking the farm to switch to a different crop. They are providing a life for their families. They can send their kids to college now and pay their mortgages. For most farming families, it is difficult, but they do it. If we want farmers to start growing more specialty crops, we need to lower the risk involved in growing fruits, vegetables, and nuts. Farmers are business people. Too much risk means they will not make the investment. Fruits and vegetables are perishable. Peaches will not last as long as the grain that can sit in a big silo for an extended period of time. That makes them a riskier investment.

As policy makers and citizens, we need to figure out how to lower the risk for fruits and vegetables just as we lowered the risk for soy, wheat, and corn. How can we stabilize prices for them? How can we build a transportation system that meets the needs that these new crops demand?

If we want healthy, local food, we need to increase demand for fruits and vegetables. Not abroad, but right here at home. We have so many public schools, colleges, and universities sprinkled throughout our country. Each of these is a market just waiting to be tapped by our local farmers. We need our children and students to eat healthy because our health system will collapse if current trends continue. So, why not open these markets more directly to our farmers? Ohio State University, for example, has more than 60,000 students. I'm sure the farmers of central Ohio would be excited about directly supplying that population with fresh, healthy, local food that was just a short drive from the farm.

While some of the corporate farms are happy to preserve the current system, which is rigged in their favor, most of the farmers I know would be more than willing to help solve these great health challenges with a new approach. And, as always, my door will be open to help piece all the necessary groups and organizations together to make this revolution happen.

Like the Millers, Peter Volz is a farmer who's working to bring fresh food to his community through a number of innovative methods. For many years, he grew vegetables in a community garden plot and was active in the community garden leadership in his hometown. In 2007, in his late 50s, he left a university job and took the big leap and started Oxford Gardens, a 4-acre market farm in Niwot, Colorado, just outside of Boulder. Peter has a small-scale polyculture farm. Polyculture, by contrast with industrial plant-growing, uses many different crops on the same soil, which mimics the diversity we find in natural ecosystems and avoids large stands of single crops. Yes, 4 acres is a tiny farm by American standards, but a lot of 4- and 5- and 6- and 20- and 40-acre farms start to add up to a significant addition to our food system.

When I visited Peter's farm, it was late spring, and as sometimes happens in the flatlands at the foothills of the Rocky Mountains, the sun was beating down on us pretty intensely, with only a light breeze. Peter's manager and four other people, several of them volunteers from Willing Workers on Organic Farms (WWOOF), were working in the rows. Even Peter was bending over and weeding, even though he spends most of his time dealing with his commercial customers, the office work, and being the face of Oxford Gardens at the farmers' market. He tries as much as possible to spend some time in the field, though. Farming is a hands-on business, to be sure.

The land he leases sits on an elbow-shaped bend in Left Hand Creek. As he walked me around the land, I sunk down a good six inches into the fine crumbly alluvial soil—excellent for vegetables. (But of course, having this kind of fine soil deposited by rivers also means you're prone to flooding. Farmers face more risks than a Wall Street trader. Mother Nature can be a pretty strict parent!)

Oxford Gardens has built a solid reputation as a reliable source of "hand-crafted" vegetables. They offer 30 different types of vegetables in more than 100 different varieties. They are not certified organic, but they follow many of the same practices as organic farms and do not use pesticides or chemical sprays of any kind.

Over the past seven years Peter and his team have become a force in both the Boulder community and now in Denver, as well. They have become a reliable supplier to more than 20 of the best restaurants in these towns of the growing, vibrant, and beautiful state of Colorado. They work the farmers' market weekly in Boulder and have built a great following with their Community Supported Agriculture (CSA) program where they build relationships between their customers and the farm. In a CSA, the customer buys the groceries before they're grown—providing the farmers with funds they need to buy seed and other important components of the farming process—and then the farm supplies them with high-quality veggies and herbs during the peak growing season. The consumer gets fresh vegetables in the spring, summer, and fall. And as they say on their website, people are "receiving produce that barely a few hours earlier was growing in the field," which is certainly preferable, since "the average produce in the grocery store is 7–14 days old and has traveled hundreds, sometimes thousands, of miles."

> "The average produce in the grocery store is 7–14 days old and has traveled hundreds, sometimes thousands, of miles."
>
> —PETER VOLZ

Oxford Gardens is also one of 13 farms that hosts open-air banquets through Meadow Lark Farm Dinners. There are farm-dinner small businesses all over America now, where chefs drive a mobile kitchen out to the farm, cook using ingredients picked that day, and serve the food, usually with wines that have been suggested (or supplied in certain jurisdictions, depending on the state's liquor laws). Diners sit at a table, often with nice tablecloths, plates, and cutlery, and experience a feast in the open air. In this case, farm-to-table is a matter of a few feet. I would just love to see this happen as part of a food education program for kids (minus the wine), where the food cost could be underwritten by a foundation, with a little help from the government.

Oxford Gardens is hot, and not just from the beating sun. Demand for their product is rapidly increasing. Their gross income increased 22 percent each year from 2009 to 2013. Even as I was corresponding with Peter about this book, he was getting requests for more business. Much of it he has to turn down.

You may also remember the huge flood that hit Colorado in September 2013. Oxford Gardens lost a substantial portion of its crop. Yet, they saw a whopping 25 percent increase over their 2012 sales. Now, they are implementing an expansion of operations that will double sales by 2016. Peter loves to quote a Chinese saying that sums up Oxford Gardens' approach to growing: "A bad farmer grows weeds. A good farmer grows crops. But the best farmer grows soil."

III

ALL WORTH IT ON THE FARM

When I was talking with Peter about all of the challenges he faces as a small farmer, including variations in rainfall, fluctuations in temperature, lack of good irrigation year-round, and the possibility of a natural disaster striking, I kept thinking about how hard it is to do this work. The people who strive to make fresh food available for us dedicate their lives to the effort. But when I asked Peter why he keeps at this Sisyphean task, he gave an answer that made it all clear:

"I had a mother come to the market with her six-year-old daughter last Saturday. We've been selling some cucumbers from our Denver greenhouse partners, and this lady has been giving them to her kids. She told me the first thing her daughter requests when she wakes up is 'Cucumber, Mommy.'

"Corny, but I hear it all the time: 'My kids never liked carrots from the regular supermarket. Now I can't give them enough of yours. They actually eat salads now!!!' I have seen kids grow up from infancy who come to the market with their parents, love good vegetables, and are healthy and beautiful. I am constantly posting kids eating vegetables on our Facebook, and they are always the most popular item."

IIIIIIIIIIIIIIIIIIIIIIIIIIIIIIIIIIIIIIIIIIIIIIIIIIIIIIIIIIIIIIIIIIIIIIIIIIIIIIIIIIIIIIIIIIIIIIIIIIIIIIIIIIIIIIIII

I just love how these farmers have a laser focus on doing what is best for the soil and for the animal, because they believe that's what's best for the consumer. They reap what they sow. There are many Millers and Volzes all across America, and they need our support— in Washington, in state governments, and at the market. Because without a market, a farmer won't be in business for long.

Meeting Michael Pollan is like experiencing a cool breeze on a sticky, hot summer day. He is a kind, refreshing presence, and his intelligence gently wakes you up. I met him for lunch at Chez Panisse, the restaurant started by Alice Waters that serves local and organic food, as well as grass-fed beef, and

> **"Buy your snacks at the farmers' market."**
>
> —MICHAEL POLLAN

celebrates the work of local farmers. Almost everything they serve is grown using sustainable farming practices. Michael is the smartest and most articulate person in the room when it comes to what we need to do to revolutionize our food system. We talked over a long lunch about food, politics, and the impact of the millennial generation. I walked away inspired by his quiet optimism about what the future of food can be. I share his optimism and know there is a movement waiting to be built that can change some of this. And Michael Pollan has been talking about this for many years.

According to Michael, the best way to help farmers move the system in a more sustainable and non-GE direction is to create markets for their products. No fuss, no cumbersome government program, just good old-fashioned free enterprise. Some of these markets are already open to non-genetically modified products, and farmers actually get a premium. In *Modern Farmer*, a forward-looking magazine that started publishing in 2013, I read an article titled "The Post-GMO Economy" where it said that "Clarkson Grain, which buys conventional and organic corn and soybeans, pays farmers a premium—up to $2 extra per bushel over the base commodity price of soybeans, $1 for corn." These products are shipped to the European Union, South Korea, and Japan, markets that look poorly upon GE crops.

And what the godfather of the good food movement is asking is, why can't we create markets right here in the United States for our farmers to sell non-GMO crops, too? And why can't we create markets for grass-fed beef, which has less total fat, saturated fat, cholesterol, and calories, and more vitamin E, beta-carotene, vitamin C, and a number of health-promoting fats, including omega-3 fatty acids and conjugated linoleic acid (CLA)?

Domestic markets for domestically produced healthy food. No global price fluctuations. No commodities needing to be traded. No futures markets. Just a farmer, some product, and a local market to sell it. And if we can correct our subsidy system, these cutting-edge farmers wouldn't be at such a disadvantage. We can level the playing field, so the market can work properly. As Melissa from Miller's Farm said, "If we didn't subsidize corn so much, the beef with hormones and antibiotics in it wouldn't be so cheap, so that McDonald's couldn't sell a hamburger for $1. Why is bad food cheap? Because the inputs are cheap." On a level playing field, with good strategies to open markets, both here and abroad, we can send these farmers into a virtuous growth spurt that can improve our health, improve our environment, and bring needed jobs and investment to our rural communities.

At a meeting in my office with four local farmers from Ohio, they were all open to switching the crops they currently produce to other crops so long as there is a market for them to sell to. As I saw up close with my visit to the Millers and Peter Volz (as well as many other farmers over the years), it's a very tough business, and almost every single farmer is carrying loans and mortgages and equipment leases. They will work longer hours and more days than anyone in America, but they need a viable market to support their operations.

A few farmers, a growing number in fact, have been finding markets—like the Millers selling to Catullo's and Peter Volz selling to a bunch of restaurants, a CSA, and the farmers' market. But the big question is how to find a lot more markets for a lot more people. Will we continue to have a small amount of high-quality food available to the elites? Hopefully not. So, how can we develop these markets? And how can we give the farmers the support they need to grow and raise the kind of food we need to be healthy?

IIIIIIIIIIIIIIIIIIIIIIIIIIIIIIIIIIIIIIIIIIIIIIIIIIIIIIIIIIIIIIIIIIIIIIIIIIIIIIIIIIIIIIIIIIIIIIIIIIIIIIIIIIIIIIIIIIIIIIIIIIIIIIIIIIII

A CASE STUDY IN AGRICULTURAL TECHNOLOGY: PURE SENSE—NEW TECHNOLOGIES TO ENHANCE AGRICULTURAL RESOURCE MANAGEMENT

Just planting gardens will not be enough to get us from where we are today to where we need to be in the future. We have to make technology work for us. This means, with support from the USDA, investing in new technologies that can scale up sustainable farming, while stopping investments in technologies that simply support the status quo of our failing food system. The kinds of technologies I am talking about are for precision irrigation, conservation, biopesticides, low-energy systems, soil remediation, land replacement technology, vertical farms, and many others. An exploration of new technologies for sustainable farming would make an entire book in itself, but I want to give you a small taste of what is possible.

Pure Sense is a California company that has installed field-monitoring stations for more than 700 customers with more than 4,000 fields that cover 300,000 acres of land in the American West. The field-monitoring sensors deliver data on moisture levels of the soil, wind, temperature, irrigation status, how much water is getting applied, and how much is actually getting to the crop. It then delivers this information wirelessly to the farmer. It uses both hardware and software to reduce nutrient runoff and the wastage of water. Farmers have more information to make better decisions.

What does this really mean for the farmer and the environment? More than 500 fields where Pure Sense was used were analyzed in 2010–2011, and water savings averaged 16 percent and energy savings averaged 12 percent. This is why this company received the California Agriculture Game Changer of the Year Award in 2011.

This is why we need to invest in new technologies like the Pure Sense monitoring system. An approach like this is supported by farmers and environmentalists alike. The people at Pure Sense think if they could take these savings and apply them to the four million acres of specialty crops in California, we could save two million acre-feet of water and 885,000 megawatts of energy per year, increase agricultural yield by 10 percent, create 2,000 jobs in California, and increase revenue by $2.5 billion.

We have to be realistic. If we're going to shift our food consumption to regional farming, we need to upgrade the technology to scale it up—to make it efficient in the short term without inflicting the long-term damage to our environment that industrial agriculture delivers. We need technologies to help us conserve water and protect and replenish our soil. Let's move some of the engineers and scientists from monoculture and pesticide research to the polyculture crop technology side of things. Smart technology will put a rocket booster on the real food revolution!

One way is to support local nonprofits like Intervale. A good friend of mine, Chuck Lief, tipped me off to this group because he was chair of their board when he lived in Vermont. He is now president of Naropa University and is a very savvy businessperson who puts his business acumen to use for social causes. As he explained it to me, the people who started Intervale wanted to get farmers to switch crops and grow more local, whole, and organic foods. But the farmers always resisted because they did not feel they had a market to sell to, and they still had mortgages and loans to pay back to keep their business afloat.

Chuck said Intervale begins its work by first talking to people who could be potential customers to create some demand for the farmers' would-be new, healthier product. They visit hospitals, colleges, schools, and restaurants to persuade them to agree to buy a certain volume of produce from the farm. Once they piece together enough demand, they go to the local banks and get them to loan the farmer money to transition to the new crop. Bingo! With that support, farmers have little reason to say no, so they're off and running. I'm sure it is not without its bumps in the road, but this is the direction we need to move in.

One of Intervale's other innovative programs is the Food Hub, an online local food market that provides year-round delivery. It builds relationships with farmers and food processors and helps build the local economy for healthy food and healthy farms. Their Farm Program helps to remove barriers to market entry for start-up farmers, such as access to land, capital, and training. They share their knowledge of equipment operation and maintenance. By leasing land, equipment, greenhouses, irrigation, and storage facilities, they help incubate new farmers and help them grow. They help keep the rent lower for new farmers, assist them in creating business plans, and provide ongoing mentorship.

I feel that part of rebalancing our national agriculture policy is to do whatever it takes to massively expand not-for-profits like Intervale. We have some programs that currently could make this happen, but they get very little money. Just imagine if we had more Intervales sprinkled in regions across America. In less than a decade we could have a good many farms converted to sustainable local farming that produce the kinds of food that keep us healthy and productive. This also keeps money and investments in our local economy: local farming, local jobs, and local control that meet the needs of the local community. No unruly government program, just strategic investments that can change the trajectory of a local food system and, in turn, our national system as well.

> "You've got to know your food to conquer your health."
>
> —VANI HARI

We can also create demand for farmers in other innovative, 21st-century ways. We need to find a way to get universities to buy food from local, regional, sustainable farms. We need to persuade the big chains that sell us our food to make more high-quality food available. Luckily some small progress is happening on this front. After years of pressure, Walmart announced in April 2014 that it would be partnering with Wild Oats to provide more affordable organic food in its stores. There is some concern that the largest retailer in the world selling organic will lead to a degrading of the quality standards for organic, but overall this is a step in the right direction, and it came about because consumers and their advocates let the company know what they wanted.

Consider Vani Hari, the Food Babe, whose story you will hear more about on the next page. If we're going to create widespread markets for better food, we're going to have to bring the campaign to that string of chain restaurants on the strips outside every city and town. She's doing that.

In 2011, she wrote a piece calling out Chick-fil-A about the harmful ingredients in their sandwiches. She rallied support from her troops and received widespread national publicity, which caused Chick-fil-A executives to invite her to their headquarters in Atlanta. In late 2013 Chick-fil-A announced that they were removing dyes, artificial corn syrup, and—in a huge win for all consumers—they said that in the next five years they would only use antibiotic-free chickens. Chick-fil-A sold 282 million chicken sandwiches in 2010. In a few years, those will all be free of antibiotics, which means of course that they will have to come from farms that raise chickens without antibiotics.

She also took on Chipotle, which has been a very progressive company where food sourcing is concerned. (I encourage you to take a look at their video on YouTube called "Back to the Start." It's got a great Willie Nelson soundtrack, and I love the message.) But the Food Babe is out to keep everyone on their toes, no matter how progressive they've been. So, she started to bug Chipotle about exactly what was in their food. She kept at it with

Making a Difference: Vani Hari, the Food Babe

Vani Hari started out just leading a pretty standard life: she went to college, got a degree, and then got a job. She worked long hours and traveled a lot, which meant that her diet was built around what she could find on the road or around the office. What that meant is that she was eating pretty poorly. This was fine for a while, but soon she started getting sick, which is what kick-started her life as the Food Babe.

She began researching food to find out what's really in it, and she began her blog, Food Babe, to chronicle what she was learning. Her amazing website now has four million unique visitors each month, who go there to learn how they can eat the way they want to eat. She is one of the foremost healthy food advocates in America and has racked up a few heavy-duty success stories, including getting giant corporations—including Kraft, Subway, Chipotle, and Chick-fil-A—to take toxic ingredients out of their products.

Her deeply researched posts, interviews, and articles have gained the respect of her audience, so that they feel empowered to take action—in the form of boycotts, protests, and petition signing. This is what brings about those impressive successes. But her activism doesn't stop at corporations; it also extends into the political realm. In 2012, she was an elected delegate to the Democratic National Convention. During Secretary of Agriculture Tom Vilsack's speech, she stood at the front of the convention center holding signs that read, "Label GMOs!" This brought national attention to a very big issue.

calls, e-mails, and even visits to local stores. One worker accidently gave her some information and she found out that there were preservatives, genetically modified organisms, and trans-fats in their food. She posted all of this information on her website. Chipotle called and tried to explain to her that for secrecy reasons, she couldn't release it. The Food Babe didn't like that and started an online petition. That got their attention and a short time later they made public all of their ingredients, another move that will ultimately help to open markets for producers of healthy food.

Kraft knows who the Food Babe is, too. After finding out that Kraft had potentially harmful food dyes Yellow 5 and Yellow 6 in their macaroni and cheese—but only in America—she started a petition. There are over 350,000 people who have signed and have stopped buying Kraft products because of this.

Subway is also feeling the heat. Here is the petition letter that over 100,000 people have signed.

Dear CEO Fred DeLuca, Head of Global Marketing Jeff Larson, and Director of Operations Joe Chaves, Subway:

> Azodicarbonamide is a chemical used "in the production of foamed plastics." It's used to make sneaker soles and yoga mats. It's also used in almost all of your Subway sandwiches, is banned across the globe, and the World Health Organization has linked it to respiratory issues, allergies, and asthma. Some studies show that when heated, azodicarbonamide turns into a carcinogen.
>
> We ask you to remove azodicarbonamide from all Subway sandwiches, and make your

bread just like you do in other countries. We deserve the same safer food our friends get overseas.

We want to really "eat fresh," not yoga mat.

Boom! This is how we build a revolution!

■ ■ ■

WHAT YOU CAN DO

One of the biggest things you can do to support the farm-to-table movement is simply to buy the products that these producers are making available. If the demand goes up, there will be more opportunities for people to move into production. With the Internet and smartphone apps, there are a lot of easy-to-access, free resources to use. The app Farm Stand (www.farmstandapp.com) can help you find a farmers' market in the U.S., U.K., Australia, or New Zealand. The organization Local Harvest (www.localharvest.org) put together a searchable database of small farms, farmers' markets, and community supported agriculture (CSA) programs that you can join. Plus there are dozens of other apps and websites, so explore and figure out what's right for you!

You can also use the USDA National Farmers Market Directory (search.ams.usda.gov/farmersmarkets), a listing of more than 8,000 farmers' markets (and growing!). Simply enter your zip code to see all the markets within a specified radius. The database is also searchable by a variety of characteristics, including what types of products are offered.

Are you someone who would consider becoming a farmer, or do you know someone? There are many great resources online to help you get started. For example, www.beginningfarmers.org has links to all sorts of resources that will help you figure out the next step for everything from finding available land to getting funding to subscribing to good agriculture magazines and newsletters. They also provide a handy quiz that can open your eyes to some of the things you may have to face if you make the choice to be a farmer. Do you have what it takes? Find out at www.beginningfarmers.org/the-beginning-farmer-quiz-do-you-have-what-it-takes.

Another good resource for learning how to farm is the Stone Barns Center for Food and Agriculture in the lower Hudson Valley in upstate New York. The center offers volunteer, internship, and apprenticeship opportunities for aspiring farmers. Find out more at www.stonebarns center.org/about-us/opportunities/index.html.

Willing Workers on Organic Farms is a network of organizations (WWOOF) worldwide that connect people who want to live and learn on organic farms and small farms with people who are looking for volunteer help. WWOOF hosts offer food, accommodation, and opportunities to learn about organic lifestyles. Volunteers give hands-on help in return. Learn more at www.wwoof international.org.

Do whatever you can to elevate the profession of farming to a higher status in this country. Make sure farmers are included in career days at your school. Talk to your kids about the importance of the work they do. Make sure those around you understand what it takes for food to get to your table.

There are young people in the Future Farmers of America who are very enthusiastic about the new way of food. Check out the Facebook page for the FFA members for 100 percent organic, ecologically respectful, sound agriculture at www.facebook.com/FfaMembersForOrganic SustainableAgriculture.

Know Your Farmer, Know Your Food (KYF2) is a program being managed by the United States Department of Agriculture. According to their website (www.usda.gov/ knowyourfarmer), their mission is to "support the critical connection between farmers and consumers and to strengthen USDA's support for local and regional food systems." They have great information about funding opportunities, plus they have other tools that can help connect you with your local agriculture purveyors. In fact, they maintain a list of food hubs, organized by state, so you can see what's available in your area (www .ams.usda.gov/AMSv1.0/getfile?dDocName=STELPR DC5091437).

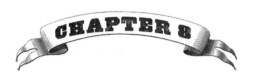

AN URBAN
FOOD REVIVAL

More than 80 percent of us live in cities now, and many of our cities are not bearing up under the strain. They need renewal and revival. Fortunately, one of the greatest ways to uplift the character of a city is to bring in more fresh food, at open markets and in urban farms. That's starting to happen in a big way, and we need it to happen in a much bigger way.

> *When we understand the connection between the food on our table and the fields where it grows, our everyday meals can anchor us to nature and the place where we live.*
>
> —ALICE WATERS

One thing that constantly impresses me about the real food revolution is that its impact will be felt in all corners of our country. When we think of food and farming, we mostly think of rural America. Commercials portray the wholesomeness of country living and use nostalgic pictures of days gone by to sell their manufactured, heavily processed food. But there is a changing perception about how a restructured food system can breathe new life into *urban* America. I see it happening in little pockets all over our country, and now it's time to fire up this part of our movement. The "fields" that Alice Waters is talking about can be, and increasingly are, very near where people live, and we need to see much more of that—not just for upper-middle-class foodies, but for everyone. An urban food revival can be a key element in urban renewal altogether. An exciting urban farming agenda can energize our cities by bringing needed investments and job creation to these hard-pressed areas while also providing the needed healthful food that will prevent illness.

One of the biggest things that has happened in the urban food landscape—and in some rural places—is the introduction of farmers' markets. These are fantastic for consumers, who get fresh food, and producers, who can cut out several layers of middlemen. And farmers' markets have taken care of some of the food deserts we talked about before. The campaign to develop these markets is going so well in some places that the opportunities for new locations are starting to become limited and farmers can only get to so many locations—New York City has 140 markets now, and is still growing!

One of my favorite experiences going to a farmers' market was in February 2014, when my friend Peter

Good, a landscape designer and builder who has lived in San Francisco for almost 35 years, took me to the oldest farmers' market in San Francisco, the Alemany Farmers' Market, which started in 1943 as a wartime measure.

To be in San Francisco is one of the more breathtaking experiences a person can have. The view from the Golden Gate Bridge over the bay is something every American should see at least once. Watching the sunlight dance on the choppy waters while the cool wind blows in my hair stops time for me. Every time I'm there I realize why people went out West to visit and never returned home. This market had the same effect on me.

The Alemany Farmers' Market sits in a low spot in the shadow of the intersection of routes 280 and 101. You drop down into it off of one of those famous San Francisco hills in the Bernal Heights neighborhood. Pete has been going to Alemany for as long as he can remember. He and his brother John, a physician in Oakland, go there every Saturday to pick up fresh fruits and vegetables for the week. The center of the market is long and wide, with about 15 stalls lining each side. Joe Montana would strain his arm throwing a football the length of this place. It's the perfect spot for strolling around on a Saturday morning.

Pete is like the mayor of the Alemany market. He knows most of the farmers and vendors there and introduced me to many of them. He knows which farmers have the best oranges, strawberries, or almonds—a good turn of events for me. It was fascinating to speak with the farmers and hear the stories involved in the seemingly simple process of setting up a booth at a space in a big city and selling produce. Most of the farms are second- or third-generation family businesses. These folks *love* their farms and love providing people with good, healthy food. To come from rural northern California and arrive in San Francisco in time for the market, they have to leave the farm at about 3 A.M. They come early, set up, interact with customers all day, and then load up and head home. It's tough work, but not one of them complained. When they weren't hawking their wares, the farmers were joking around with the customers and teasing their competitors about whose product was better. Farmers' teenage children were working some of the stalls, often half-asleep behind the counters. Getting up that early is not generally on a teenager's agenda.

As we walked around, I couldn't help but take pictures for my wife. She loves going to the farmers' market, and this would have really pleased her. She would have gone crazy at the high piles of leafy vegetables and the riot of color in the bins of root vegetables. We tasted everything that was out: walnuts, almonds, grapefruit, cantaloupe, olives, olive oil, and cheese. And then, we hit the mother lode—honey! I know, honey *is* sugar, but the real stuff is so flavorful, it's like fine wine. You savor it; you don't gorge on it. As I said earlier, I'll never stop appreciating the magical process whereby the honey takes on the characteristics of the flowers the bees pollinate. Jan C. Snyder, who is 80 if he's a day, was selling every different kind of honey you could imagine, as well as bee pollen and royal jelly. And I purchased a jar of each flavor. Orange blossom, alfalfa, sage; you name it, he had it. My wife and I love to put a little honey in our coffee or tea in the morning. Or I'll have a little spoonful before a workout. This honey disappeared rather quickly once I got back to Ohio, and when I asked my wife where it all went, she said, "Your boy here can't walk past the cupboard without taking a fingerful of it." Alfalfa is Mason's favorite, and he's got to do a little work on the savoring-versus-gorging thing. On the other hand, maybe he's developing some discrimination, because one day Andrea came into the kitchen to find Mason and his friend Albert sitting in front of five open jars of honey, doing comparison tasting!

There aren't any junk food or souvenir vendors at Alemany. It's simply a great outdoor market with good food. Its fans call it "the people's market" for its reasonable prices and to distinguish it from the huge market downtown by the bay, which is a bit of a tourist trap.

I can hear some of you saying that while this sounds great for California, other places don't have its climate and growing season. But there were farmers' markets in Pennsylvania and Ohio long before Alemany showed up in San Francisco. The Lancaster Central Market is the oldest continuously operating market in the country, having been incorporated right into the city's design in the 18th century. Cincinnati's Findlay Market, the oldest in Ohio, dates back to 1855. These old markets have many new friends now. Happily, the USDA started keeping track of farmers' market growth starting in 1994. There's been a healthy increase: from fewer than 2,000 in 1994, there are now more than 8,000, and counting. I'd love to see this number double in the next few years.

And I love the reforms in food stamp programs that my friend and colleague Representative Marcia Fudge is pushing. Marcia is a representative from Cleveland and chair of the Congressional Black Caucus. She is a tenacious and innovative leader who knows the importance of getting healthy food into our urban centers. She pushes ideas like expanding the Supplemental Nutrition Assistance Program benefits when they're used to buy fresh produce at a farmers' market. These are the kinds of innovative solutions we need to support if we're to grow markets for our local farmers and help get rid of the food deserts that lead to obesity and ill health.

> "It is a lot cheaper to feed [people in need] and give them good nutrition than it is to take care of them on the other end."
>
> —REP. MARCIA FUDGE

Another effort that is helping address a lack of food in urban centers is actually based on growing food in our cities. And I'm proud to say that the upper Midwest has become a hotbed (and a seedbed) for innovative urban agriculture projects. There are important programs in Milwaukee, Chicago, Cleveland, and Youngstown, plus so many more. Detroit in particular has made some real strides in this area. This town used to have a population of 1.9 million; now it's 700,000. They have 30,000 acres of distressed land in the city. These are pretty challenging times, but over the past few years Detroit has seen a number of urban growers and farmers begin to transform the city, including a Whole Foods urban program that I will discuss in the next chapter. The heartland is leading the way in urban agriculture in many ways. (Okay, so that's some serious regional pride, I know, but what can I say? I dig my bioregion.)

If we're going to drive ag investment into our urban areas, we need to turn old dilapidated neighborhoods into vibrant centers of production, just like they've been doing in Detroit. And I don't believe we need any new money to do this. We simply need to shift some of the money that's going to make bad food cheap and use it to increase production in our urban areas. Plus we need to make laws and policies easier to navigate. Interestingly, Peter Good, the same friend who took me to the Alemany Farmers' Market, has helped two of San Francisco's urban ag innovators, Brooke Budner and Caitlyn Galloway, install an irrigation system at Little City Gardens, the small farm they established in the Mission Terrace neighborhood. Budner and Galloway were instrumental in causing the city to abolish restrictive zoning laws that inhibited the setting up of urban farms, and Little City Garden folk—along with many others urban farmers—successfully fought for the passage of California's AB551, which incentivizes the use of private land for urban ag, by allowing urban land where food is grown to be taxed at a lower rate.

The biggest mover and shaker I can think of in the urban ag movement, however, is Will Allen—he's like the head coach of urban farming. I met Will a few years back when he came to Youngstown to teach and inspire the people leading our urban ag efforts. He's a former professional basketball player, and he's super tall with a huge smile and a cool, engaging demeanor. He's a no-nonsense guy who will not sugarcoat the fact that it takes hard work and grit to make a farm work in an urban area. He was the son of a sharecropper and the first African American to play basketball at the University of Miami, so he knows how to face difficult odds and bring about change. He was one of *Time* magazine's top 100 most influential people in the world in 2010, and has been honored by the Clinton Global Initiative. He's also a MacArthur Foundation fellow and one of the first people to show how urban farming can be a catalyst for growth in hard-hit cities like Milwaukee.

Growing Power, Inc., his nonprofit, supports communities in their efforts to grow safe, high-quality, affordable food. In addition to its inner-city farm, it has a 40-acre farm west of Milwaukee in Merton, Wisconsin; a project in Chicago run by his daughter Erika; and satellite training sites in Arkansas, Georgia, Kentucky, Massachusetts, Cleveland, and Mississippi. Altogether, Growing Power houses 20,000 plants and vegetables, and thousands of fish, chickens, goats, ducks, rabbits, and bees.

> "If we can make small farming economically viable again, and if we can involve young people in this work, we can go a long way in teaching lessons of character that will produce more resilient and capable citizens."
>
> —WILL ALLEN

It all began when Will retired, first from basketball and then from a corporate career, and took over responsibility for running his wife's family farm. In 1993, he went looking for a place to sell his produce in the city and stumbled upon a garden center with an adjacent three acres that turned out to be the last tract of land in Milwaukee still zoned for agriculture. As he began to work the land there, something wonderful happened: neighborhood kids, including some who lived in the largest low-income public housing project in Milwaukee, began to ask him for advice and assistance with growing their own vegetables. He saw that teaching and training people in the neighborhoods to farm empowered them and helped to develop food security: supplying healthy food at affordable prices. Growing Power, which now has a staff of 65, has three main areas of focus:

1. In their six greenhouses, year-round hoop houses (structures that create a controlled growing environment, much like a greenhouse), and animal pens—and in their satellite locations—they demonstrate high-yield growing methods they've developed that can work in urban environments, using composting, vermiculture (using worms to enrich soil), and aquaponics (growing fish and food plants in a closed system).

2. They provide education and technical assistance worldwide for people who want to develop the skills to replicate what they're doing.

3. They're a substantial producer and distributor of produce, grass-based meats, and value-added products. They supply many restaurants and small grocery stores in Milwaukee, Madison, and Chicago. The Rainbow Farmers Cooperative they started gives a leg up to 300 small family farms across the United States in finding reliable markets for their products.

Will's organization has gone far beyond being a local initiative. It's a national (and even international) resource for city dwellers, including many underprivileged people, that enables them to make a transition from being a consumer to a producer. When he visited Youngstown, he talked with us, among other things, about "food racism." In a similar way that banks redline poor neighborhoods, African American and Latino neighborhoods are denied wholesome food. He gave us the gospel of urban agriculture with the fervor of a preacher. I get really pumped up by that. Tilling soil, bending over plants, deepening our connection to the land and the animals that sustain us, feeding others— these can be deeply spiritual acts. In some ways, the food revolution is a revolution of the spirit.[3]

About the same time that Will Allen was setting up his organization, Les Brown, of the Chicago Coalition for the Homeless, set up Growing Home, in that city. Now run by Harry Rhodes (since Brown passed away in 2005), the organization operates a training program for homeless people to work at three sites: the Wood Street Urban Farm, the Su Casa Market Garden, and the Les Brown Memorial Farm in Marseilles, 75 miles south of the city. The produce is sold at a farmers' market in downtown Chicago and at on-site farm stands. It's also served in top Chicago restaurants and distributed in weekly food baskets through a CSA.

Rhodes is a founding member of the Chicago-based Advocates for Urban Agriculture, and he's very upbeat about the future of urban agriculture. In particular, he sees it as offering educational opportunities and a means of turning lives around. He told a reporter, "Experiential education can make a big difference. It helps people see food in ways they haven't before. When people come to

---

3   Will and I clearly see eye to eye, since he titled his 2012 memoir *The Good Food Revolution,* a poignant account of how he came to be a leader in this movement.

our farm stand in the inner city, or an open house, or a cooking workshop, they have a hands-on experience. Slowly attitudes change. Our graduates are different people than when they started. Not long ago, one of them said, 'When I first came here, I didn't even know how a vegetable grew. Now I'm growing my own.'"

> "There's nothing like working in the soil to give you roots and a sense of belonging."
>
> —HARRY RHODES

In Cleveland, the Rid-All Green Partnership operates an urban farm and educational center right in the heart of one of Cleveland's toughest neighborhoods. I visited it in the spring of 2014 and met Damien Forshe, one of three childhood friends who grew up in the old Kinsman neighborhood, a part of Cleveland known as the Forgotten Triangle. They've now returned to transform it. I toured their place with him and Marc White, their site manager and head farmer. I was blown away. As eight or nine young kids played basketball across the street, they laid out their vision for where they want to take Rid-All, which is one of Growing Power's regional training centers.

Rid-All has three acres, two greenhouses, and four hoop houses, and plans to expand across the street. In addition to growing fruit and vegetables, they make compost for their own land and to sell to local partners, and they raise tilapia. They run the greenhouses and hoop houses in the winter by mixing piles of compost full of beer waste (they make their own beer, too!), coffee grinds, and wood chips. The combination creates a

Making a Difference: Will Allen, Bringing Farming to the City

Will Allen, at 6'7", agile and muscular, was perfectly suited for basketball. He helped take his team to the state championship at Richard Montgomery High School in Rockville, Maryland, where his parents had a small vegetable farm and adjacent house allotted to them by the woman who employed his mother as a domestic servant. Both his parents had lived in South Carolina as sharecroppers, tenant farmers who gave up half their crop in return for the right to pick it. In his book, *The Good Food Revolution*, Allen recalls, "I didn't like the work of planting and harvesting that I was made to do as a child . . . I fought my family's history. Yet the desire to farm hid inside me."

After becoming the first black player at the University of Miami, he went on to have a short career in the American Basketball Association, and overseas. At 28, he left basketball and moved to Milwaukee, his wife's hometown, and eventually to her family's farm outside the city. While working as a star salesman, he began farming before and after work. One day, on a sales run for Procter & Gamble, he passed a derelict greenhouse with a FOR SALE sign near Milwaukee's largest public housing project. Not long after, at 44, he left his job. He was competitive and proud of his accomplishments in business, but work was "a project of my wallet rather than a project of my heart."

Allen nurtured his funky greenhouse into Growing Power, now an internationally recognized innovator in urban farming. "The work of my adult life," Allen says, "has been to heal the rift in our food system," which puts healthy food and the income from growing it out of reach of the disadvantaged, and "to create alternative ways of growing and distributing fresh food."

biomolecular reaction inside so it heats the pile to 150 degrees and keeps the inside of the houses warm.

In Youngstown, millions of dollars from the Neighborhood Stabilization Program (NSP), a granting program managed by the U.S. Department of Housing and Urban Development, have been spent to knock down 4,000 homes, focusing on the building up of a famous old neighborhood that used to be the home of Idora Park, which was an amusement park and a venue for big bands. As the steel mills closed and the city declined, this precious little amusement park and the neighborhood around it fell into a deep decline. Now, the city of Youngstown, along with the Youngstown Neighborhood Development Corporation (YNDC), have knocked down some old homes, refurbished a few others, and moved in new homeowners. YNDC, under the leadership of Presley Gillespie, the nephew of the great jazz trumpeter Dizzy Gillespie, brought some of the swing back into the Idora neighborhood. When you walk into his office, you should be prepared to be motivated either by a book he's reading or a saying he has up on his wall. He is pure inspiration. He comes out of the banking world and didn't want to run a nonprofit unless it could eventually sustain itself. He believes NGOs should use grants to help them get off the ground or supplement programming, but they need to create value by selling products or services that can keep them afloat.

One of the key elements of the Idora revival is to fill open spaces with hoop houses and raised plant beds and have kids work there in the summer as a learning experience. We were able to secure a few federal grants for YNDC, but what I love about Presley is that he drove the organization toward self-sufficiency. For example, they're growing lots of root vegetables in their lots.

Why? Because they get a premium price for them. For urban ag to work, it needs to be economically viable. If government can give a leg up by supplying funds to buy equipment, hoop houses to extend the growing season, and more land to increase yields, it can be done.

Of course, urban neighborhoods are not only deficient in agriculture. As I mentioned in chapter 4, they are also deficient in grocery stores, and particularly stores that offer fresh food. These food deserts lead to poor nutrition, and they also decrease the quality of life by decreasing opportunities for social connection. The market is not only a place to acquire food; it's a place to meet and greet. It's a center of community. The actor Wendell Pierce from the HBO series *The Wire* (where he played detective Bunk Moreland) and *Treme* (where he played trombonist Antoine Batiste) has started a grocery store in his native New Orleans, called Sterling Farms. He was motivated to do so, he says, because his hometown "was populated with food deserts and underserved communities where people didn't have access to fresh produce and fresh foods."

Pierce goes on to say that many people in America are used to hopping in the car and going to the grocery store, but for many others that means "hopping on a bus, having to walk, or having to go a little farther because they don't have one in their neighborhood. That shouldn't happen in America. So we see those neighborhoods as emerging markets instead of depressed areas. It's proving to be true."

Beyond the value of bringing more fresh food to people in underserved areas, Pierce sees great benefit in re-creating the market as a gathering place. One of his greatest memories, he says, is "as we say in New Orleans, 'making groceries' with my mother on a Friday night. It was a ritual to go there . . . Seeing the men and the women getting off work—they had a little bar and restaurant in this place—and knowing the fishmonger, knowing the butchers, and having our favorite cashier. It was the equivalent of a town square. That neighborhood grocery is something that we take for granted; we don't realize it until we lose it."

In chapter 9, I talk about Whole Foods' initiative to have a store in inner-city Detroit, because I want to highlight the food education work the company is doing there. It's also good to see people like Wendell Pierce and his partners in Sterling Farms taking on the risk involved in entering the food marketplace because they want to see their city thrive again. May there be many more markets like Sterling Farms in cities across America.

ROOFTOP GARDENS

Rooftop gardens are a great source of fresh food in the city—and an energy saver. A University of Michigan study in 2006 compared the expected costs of conventional roofs with the cost of a 21,000-square-foot (1,950 m^2) green roof and all its benefits, such as storm-water management and improved public health from the absorption of nitrogen oxides. The green roof would cost \$464,000 to install versus \$335,000 for a conventional roof in 2006 dollars. However, over its lifetime, the green roof would save about \$200,000. Nearly two-thirds of these savings would come from reduced energy needs for the building with the green roof.

A rooftop garden's key environmental benefits are impressive. Researchers estimate that a 1,000-square-foot (93 m²) green roof can remove about 40 pounds of particulate matter (PM) from the air in a year, while also producing oxygen and removing carbon dioxide (CO_2) from the atmosphere. Forty pounds of PM is roughly how much 15 passenger cars will emit in a year of typical driving.

In addition, a modeling study for Washington, DC, examined the potential air quality benefits of installing green roofs on 20 percent of total roof surface for buildings with roofs greater than 10,000 square feet (930 m²). Under this scenario, green roofs would cover about 20 million square feet (almost 2 million m²), and remove annually about six tons of ozone (O_3) and almost six tons of PM of less than 10 microns (PM10), or the equivalent of the pollutants that could be absorbed by about 25,000 to 33,000 street trees.

|||||||||||||||||||||||||||||||||||||||||||||||||||||||||||||||||||||||||||||||||||||||||||||||||||||||||||||||

One of the unexpected things that also comes from urban farming and having fresh food outlets and restaurants that serve local food is the development of regional delicacies. *Terroir* (from *terra*, Latin for "earth") is a French word usually used to refer to the environmental conditions, like soil and climate, that food is grown in that give it unique characteristics. It's mostly used when talking about grapes from a certain region that impart a character to a given wine. A Bordeaux has a certain taste based on its *terroir*. A Napa Valley cabernet or even the alfalfa honey that Mason likes is influenced by its *terroir*. I find it very exciting to think of how we can take classic American cities like Baltimore, Cleveland, Milwaukee, Detroit, Pittsburgh, Toledo, Minneapolis–St. Paul, and many others and breathe new life into them by making some key investments into their *"terroir"* and the goods that they produce.

Each of these places has a different climate, different soil, and different ways they prepare the local food they grow. Let's start celebrating these great American cities and stop looking the other way and hoping the challenges they face will simply go *poof*. For one thing, let's reclaim depressing, blighted, and crime-ridden blocks and convert them into usable land. They won't be populated again, but they can be put to good use. The federal NSP has given billions of dollars to local communities to knock down dilapidated homes, clearing entire blocks, making the way for urban agriculture projects. But for the many cities that have lost their tax base and need assistance to make way for urban ag projects, there is not enough money to go around. We need more of this type of investment if we're going to ramp up the urban farming programs to a level where they can have an impact on the local food system.

■ ■ ■

WHAT YOU CAN DO

The most direct thing you can do to spur urban farming is to start doing it yourself! Everyone can start a garden. Even if you're in an apartment and only have a window-sill or a balcony, you can grow a variety of vegetables or herbs. (Basil, parsley, tomatoes, beans, lettuce, and turnips are just a few possibilities.) Search "growing herbs in small landscapes" or "growing herbs in an apartment," and you will find some great information to get you started. It's very easy.

Before you jump in, take a look at www.urban farmonline.com, which links to a great USDA zone map and crop profiles so you can find which crop varieties would grow best in your region. It even has a calendar for when you should plant your crops!

If you don't want to start from scratch, you can take part in community gardening. The American Community Gardening Association (communitygarden.org) provides would-be gardeners with all the information they could want, including a search function that can help you find a community garden near you.

If you're interested in starting a community garden, the American Community Gardening Association website can help you there, too. It outlines steps to organize a garden committee and the tools you'll need, plus it has considerations for finding a site for your garden. It also lays out helpful items such as garden agreements that can help you establish a community garden and best practices. You can also reach out directly to your city or town. Ask your city council or town council whether there are any ordinances in place for using vacant land as temporary or permanent gardens.

The EPA has a "Brownfields Program," which gives money to develop community gardens from abandoned properties. They've had a great deal of success already, with programs in all 50 states. One is the Allen Street Community Garden in Somerville, MA. The Allen Street

Community Garden was a former contaminated zone, which has now been developed into an oasis of flowers and vegetables. The garden even has a plot accessible for disabled individuals. There are so many residents wanting to join that there are more than 25 people on the waiting list. See http://www.epa.gov/brownfields.

To get involved in a brownfields garden, check out the "Where You Live" section at the EPA brownfields website to see if there are any clean-up programs or gardens near you (http://www.epa.gov/brownfields /bfwhere.htm).

To create a brownfields site in your community:

- Contact your state environmental agency, agricultural extension office, or state brownfield team to see if they have any assessed or prospective sites that would be applicable for funding. You can find a list of useful contacts here: http://www .epa.gov/brownfields/contacts.htm.

- If you already have a site in mind (and it needs to be assessed or cleaned), you will need to have your town apply for a brownfield grant fund.

- You can go to the EPA brownfields website to learn more about the program— they even have a business plan to help you along the way: http://www.epa.gov /brownfields/urbanag/pdf/urban_farm _business_plan.pdf.

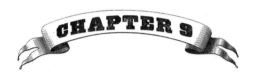

EDUCATING THE
NEXT GENERATION

Too few of our children are learning where food comes from, how it grows, what's nutritious, what's not, and what the best cooking methods are. What could be more essential to life? Thankfully, a few pioneers are getting us off to a good start.

> *There was a time when the family and the social milieu transmitted knowledge of foods, recipes, alimentary customs, and the recurring yearly occasions for special meals. Today this chain of transmission has been severed, and neither the schools nor other social institutions have taken its place.*
>
> —CARLO PETRINI

I love cooking. There is nothing better to me than being in the kitchen with my wife while we are putting a family meal together. The kids come in and help out with little tasks here or there, too, especially when dessert is involved. And the dogs also love to get a little piece of the action. Cooking and having a family meal together is a ritual that's sacred for me. I miss it so much when I'm in DC, and look forward to it when I return home.

When I hear of so many families not bothering with family dinner, it saddens me. It's important on so many levels. It's a chance for everyone to share their day and to slow down and savor the food and the company. It's also a chance for children to experience food preparation as something other than what happens behind the counter or in a back room.

This was a natural part of growing up for me. I was raised garden-to-table: from my Italian grandparents' garden just a couple of blocks from my childhood home to the table they set in their kitchen. I'd spend a lot of time down there with them during the summer, because it was a short bike ride away, and no one loves you like your grandparents. Every spring my grandfather planted tomatoes, lettuce, hot peppers, sweet peppers, zucchini, beans, and cucumbers. In the fall, he'd plant a massive amount of garlic, and we used it in or on just about everything we cooked.

There was a friendly competition between family gardens, and it was always one of the chief topics of conversation. Everyone rooted for the others to have a really good garden—just not as good as theirs. One year my grandfather Rizzi and his brother-in-law, my great-uncle Phil, were looking at his garden. Along comes my grandmother's dad, who slowly walked over to look at the garden and stand with them. My grandfather, who had a wonderful sense of humor, winked at my uncle and said to him, "Phil, they told me that each of these pepper plants would grow a bushel full of peppers this big." He put his pointing fingers about a foot apart. His father-in-law perked up and said in his thick Italian accent, "Johnny, who tell you that bullashit?" They all had a good laugh.

Watching my grandmother cook was always so much fun. We would walk out to the garden and pick veggies right off the plant. After a while, I started to know exactly what we were going to eat by what she picked. If she picked squash, we were having what she called *cagoots*: eggs, garlic, and cut-up squash cooked in a huge pan. Wow was that good. Tomatoes meant we were probably having pasta, and she would slice the tomatoes, drizzle them with olive oil, pepper, and just a little bit of oregano. If we picked lots of peppers that meant chicken and peppers cooked up with a ton of garlic and fresh bread from the local baker, who also happened to be my cousin.

My grandfather was also quite a culinary master—and his specialty was hot peps, a local delicacy that I haven't been able to find anywhere else in the country. Every year he would go to a local woman and buy a couple bushels of hot peppers. He followed a detailed and delicate process of cutting the peppers, taking the seeds out, letting them dry overnight, and filling mason jars full of them with oil, salt, and garlic. He would make enough to last the entire year. We put them on just about everything we ate or just slathered them on bread. It seems like everyone back home has his or her own recipe for hot peps. Some people use vinegar or medium-hot peppers, some use less or more, and some even add a little bit of tomato sauce. One time I was cooking ca-goots on a local morning TV show in Youngstown, and I mentioned how much I loved hot peps. People started to drop off jars of their homemade hot peps at my house and office. It was crazy how many I ended up with. I ate them all.

My cousins and uncles made wine. Some of it was very good and some was so vinegary that we put it on salads. They made their own dried sausage and sometimes beer. Everyone shared. They shared their garden, their wine, their food, and, like my constituents did for me, their hot peps. Food and cooking were the glue that held families and neighborhoods together. No one explicitly taught me about this; it was just what I saw growing up. For genera-tions, family recipes, knowledge about how to cook, and family traditions and rituals were passed down. But now because of the speed of life and our absorption in the digi-tized virtual realm, we've lost the joy of cooking and the benefits that come with doing things togeth-er as a family or a group of friends.

> **"There's nothing better than a home-cooked meal straight from the garden."**
>
> —MY GRANDFATHER JOHN RIZZI

For our health and for our well-being, I would love to see cooking make a big comeback, not because I'm nostalgic about my own childhood—although I do love remembering those spe-cial moments with my grandparents. I want to bring it back because cooking food that we grow has been a part of our cultures for 60,000 years. Cooking and eating to-gether is a tradition deep in our bones.

How do we get it back? We teach our children—and fortunately there are already some very exciting programs going on to do just this in many areas of the country.

llllllllllllllllllllllllllllllllllllllllllllllllllllllllllllllllllllllllllllllllllllllllllllllllllllllllllllllllllllll

MASSIVE FOOD MARKETING TO CHILDREN

As a new father, I'm finding out how hard it is to control the environment for Mason and Bella. I suspect it will be even harder for Brady, the newest addition to our family, as he gets older. We must talk as much as we can about healthy food and healthy habits to our kids—without turning into boring old scolds. We, as parents, are their first teachers and coaches. Unfortunately, a lot of people in the food industry do not make it easy. They aggressively market to our kids. And they market the crappiest food with the most sugar, high-fructose corn syrup, and other garbage in it. The commercials and the marketing are winning the day. We need to push back. Congress has several times asked the Institute of Medicine (IOM) to report on food marketing to children. Here are the findings from the Yale Rudd Center for Food Policy and Obesity:

Food marketing to children and adolescents is a major public health concern. According to the Rudd Center for Food Policy and Obesity at Yale University, the food industry spends $1.8 billion per year in the U.S. on marketing targeted to young people. The overwhelming majority of these ads are for unhealthy products, high in calories, sugar, fat, and/or sodium.

On television alone the average U.S. child sees approximately 13 food commercials every day, or 4,700 a year; and teens see more than 16 per day, or 5,900 in a year. The food products advertised most extensively include high-sugar breakfast cereals, fast food and other restaurants, candy, and sugary drinks. In comparison, children see about one ad per week for healthy foods, such as fruits and vegetables, and bottled water.

Companies increasingly market to young people anywhere they spend their time, including in schools, on the Internet, and on mobile phones. They continue to find new and creative ways to reach children, often blurring the line between content and advertising and encouraging children to send marketing messages to their friends through YouTube, Facebook, and other social media. Food company websites targeted to children usually contain "advergames" and other entertaining content to keep them engaged with the brands as long as possible.

The messages in youth-targeted food advertisements encourage children to pester their parents to buy the products, promote snacking between meals, and portray positive outcomes from consuming high-calorie, nutritionally poor foods. To children it appears cool, fun, and exciting to eat these unhealthy products anytime, anywhere. We've all been on the other end of these requests. Isn't parenting hard enough without having to do battle with the billion-dollar cereal industry?

There is one sign of hope, however. In 2012, the Disney corporation banned all junk food advertising during programs that cater to children—on their TV channels, radio programs, and websites. It would be great if more companies would do this type of thing.

|||||||||||||||||||||||||||||||||||||||||||||||||||||||||||||||||||||||||||||||||||||||||||||||||||||||||||||||||||||||||||||||||||||||||||||||||||||||

Alice Waters is the queen bee of the organic food movement and the genius behind Chez Panisse, the organic restaurant I had lunch at with Michael Pollan. Alice is as much a social activist as she is a chef and restaurateur. Her passion about bringing healthy food and cuisine into the world has sparked a movement we're all a part of now. She is a major advocate for the Slow Food movement, which was started in Italy (big surprise) by Carlo Petrini in 1986 to celebrate local food, protect biodiversity, and promote small-scale products in order to preserve food traditions for the next generation. Alice is an inspiring role model we can look to in taking this revolution to the next level. She advocates for every aspect of food: the economy of the farmers, the quality and taste of the food, its nutritional value, and our customs for acquiring, cooking, and eating it. One of the campaigns she speaks most fervently about today is the work she is doing for kids: the Edible Schoolyard and the School Lunch Initiative.

> "Cook together. Include your family and friends, and especially children. When children grow, cook, and serve food, they want to eat it. The hands-on experience of gardening and cooking teaches children the value and pleasure of good food almost effortlessly."
>
> —ALICE WATERS

The Edible Schoolyard project started in 1995 from a grant from the Chez Panisse Foundation to the Martin Luther King Jr. Middle School in Berkeley. This grant helped build a one-acre organic garden with an adjoining classroom that looks and functions like a kitchen. The idea was to give young kids the opportunity to learn how to grow, harvest, and cook the foods coming out of the garden. The success of the Edible Schoolyard led to the School Lunch Initiative. Alice's foundation gave a grant to the Berkeley School District in 2005 to hire a director of nutrition services (I'd like to see one of those in every school district, wouldn't you?) to bring wholesome food to the 10,000 students of the district. They were able to get rid of almost all of the processed food in the school district, they had organic veggies and fruit daily, and (check this out) they did it within the district's budget!

The Edible Schoolyard has spread, with affiliates currently in San Francisco, New York, Los Angeles, New Orleans, and Greensboro, North Carolina. Each affiliate changes the program to fit the local culture or goals of the school or community, and some are run through Boys & Girls Clubs or local museums. Schools can build it into the curriculum and use it as an opportunity to teach other subjects like science. In New Orleans, they teach the kids how to cook Creole, and also about traditions unique to the people of the bayou. (If we had a school like this in my hometown, maybe they would teach about Grandpa Rizzi's hot peps!)

When I visit schools during lunch hour and see the horrible foods kids are eating, it makes my heart sink. How can they learn on this food? And how will they learn about food without a better example? We owe it to the next generation to set them up for success. That means learning how to stay healthy and how to put food into their bodies that keeps them focused and relaxed at school. It also means learning about the magic of growing food, to see where it comes from and what makes it grow. Alice says the Edible Schoolyard is all about "transforming public education by awakening children's senses, nourishing their minds and bodies, and teaching them values that we need for the future of this planet." Amen.

Early in 2014, I was in New York City, and took the opportunity to visit another school that has a food education program. New York is brimming with such programs; there are hundreds happening all over the city.

I was fortunate to spend time with Meredith E. Hill at Columbia Secondary School for Math, Science, and Engineering in South Harlem. "Professor Hill," as her students call her, teaches English and also runs the gardening program. She greeted me by the door, and I immediately realized how lucky her students are to have her as a teacher. She is bright eyed and well educated, and radiates an excitement for her work that is infectious. She had her students do a brief presentation for me so I could see what they were up to. Before they started, I said hello to each of them and they all looked me in the eye when they shook my hand. A good sign, I thought.

I was so impressed with how strong their public speaking skills were for such young kids. (Some of them were much better than several of my colleagues on Capitol Hill, I have to say.) They stood tall and articulated their points and had a strong grasp of the material. Something very cool was going on at this school. While these kids are technically the students, they are also the teachers. The sixth, seventh, and eighth graders actually teach at workshops on composting, and have a much deeper knowledge of how to compost, what to compost, and how to grow a garden than nearly every other American. They often teach their own parents how to do these things at home.

Professor Hill gets the kids' attention with dirt and worms. Once she has them interested, she finds a way to bring the topic into her English class, so it doesn't seem disconnected from the rest of what they're learning. In one case, she had her students read the young readers edition of Michael Pollan's *The Omnivore's Dilemma*. (Everywhere I go in my exploration of the world of good food, I keep running into this guy.) Through the written word, they deepened their understanding of what

Making a Difference: Meredith Hill, Food Educator

As a child, Meredith Hill remembers spending most of her time outdoors, digging in the dirt, planting flowers, and playing by the Merrimack River in Haverhill, a small town northeast of Boston. Surrounded by farms and forests, she always loved nature and helped her mother and aunt in their flower gardens, but her favorite things to grow were all edible.

Meredith came to New York to study at Barnard College and eventually ended up getting a teaching degree, inspired by a summer she spent working in a youth program. When she started at Columbia Secondary School, she once took her class to a nearby park, where she was alarmed when they were afraid of sitting on the ground or coming in contact with bugs. She decided to reach out to her colleagues to see if there was a way to create a curriculum to allow the kids to experience the natural world. They soon started a garden on the school roof that ultimately led to developing a vacant lot into a community garden.

Meredith has now shifted the focus of her sixth-grade English class to "From the Ground Up." She is continually touched by her students' wonder at seeing things grow. As she uprooted a potted plant to put it in the ground at the garden, one of her students looked on slack-jawed. It really is magic, she thought. If children are to get a full education, she feels it's essential that they have a haven in the city—a place to connect with nature and to have an awareness of the natural world that is often easy to miss in the city.

they're doing with the compost and why they're doing it. In their reading in English class, they learn what foods are good for them, how to read labels, and what kind of chemicals may be in certain commercial fertilizers.

As far as I can tell, the kids absolutely love it. In their garden they grow kale, Swiss chard, basil, tomatoes, eggplant, and more. And they don't just learn how to dig a hole and plant a seed; they also learn how a vegetable or plant is going to interact in its environment. For example, they plant roses, daisies, and other flowers that are considered pollinator attractors—so they can attract bees to do the ever-important job of pollination. It's so exciting to see that these kids already understand how delicately interconnected our ecosystem is. They can start shaping our culture, attitudes, and our food system so we can reverse some of the current trends. What if every school used this kind of approach? We could have a generation of awake and aware citizens who, regardless of what career path they followed, would be fine examples of healthy, balanced living.

|||||||||||||||||||||||||||||||||||||||||||||||||||||||||||||||||||||||||||||||||||||||||||||||||||||||||||||||||||||||||||||||||||||||||||

FOOD REVOLUTION IN POPULAR CULTURE

In the past few years, we've seen an uptick of popularity in television programming and books that are trying to appeal to a younger generation. For example, Jamie Oliver, the lively and popular chef from the United Kingdom who is on a mission to reduce obesity and improve the health of America's children, took home an Emmy for his reality TV show *Jamie Oliver's Food Revolution* (there's that word again). He now has a campaign called "Get Food Education in Every Classroom" that is spreading across the U.S. Anyone can download the campaign's "toolkits"—called Get the Facts, Find

Support, and Start a Campaign—to get food education going in a local school.

It's also worth noting that PBS has an excellent TV show called *Hey Kids, Let's Cook!,* where nutritionist Kathy Powers cooks healthy and tasty meals with children and teens. Kathy also has a great blog on the show's website.

There has been a whole spate of cookbooks aimed at children so that they can work alongside their parents in the kitchen. These come in a number of varieties, and it seems that you can get one that will satisfy any interest—from known chefs, like Alice Waters (*Fanny at Chez Panisse*) and vegetarian chef Mollie Katzen (*Get Cooking*), to famous characters (*The Unofficial Harry Potter Cookbook*) to classic kitchen names (*Better Homes and Gardens New Junior Cookbook*).

While the means vary, the thing that all these shows and books have in common is a desire to help kids learn about where food comes from and how to eat it in a healthy way.

|||||||||||||||||||||||||||||||||||||||||||||||||||||||||||||||||||||||||||||||||||||||||||||||||||||||||||||||||||||

Another interesting education initiative was started by Whole Foods in Detroit, which located a store in the midtown area of the city. And it sounds like it's going well. Walter Robb, the co-CEO of Whole Foods said, "A lot of things we hoped would work [in Detroit] are working, and I just couldn't be more pleased with that, particularly at a time when the narrative about the city is so negative. I have to tell you, there is just a lot positive about that community."

Whole Foods is keeping their prices competitive for the area, which is good to see in and of itself, but they are also educating the public on how to choose healthy food. They have a community nutritionist who helps people find out how to eat well without going broke. They're also offering free classes on health and wellness. "We came here to confront the issues of racism and elitism," Robb said. He doesn't want Whole Foods to be pigeonholed as elitist, and the company's investment in Detroit is a good start in that direction.

It's encouraging to see that Whole Foods is active in making sure the next generation of Americans knows how to eat healthy. (Of course, they want them to become customers someday, but if they're educating them to eat fresh and healthy, I can't complain.) The Whole Kids Foundation has granted $4.2 million to 2,100 schools since 2011 with their School Garden grant program. The foundation is also superb at arming people with the information and resources they need to not only get money for their schools, but also build local coalitions in the community that are essential to a successful program.

In addition, Whole Foods has a Healthy Teachers program, which instructs teachers how to take care of themselves and also present healthy living concepts to their students. The foundation runs a two-hour course for teachers out of most of their stores! We need the innovation and ingenuity of the private sector to drive the real food revolution. I hope to see a lot more CEOs in the food sector join people like Walter Robb and John Mackey in creating markets for the kind of food we need to thrive.

There are a couple of other programs that have really caught my eye as I've been studying this topic. One is associated with the Rid-All program I talked about in the last chapter. This group is developing a memorandum of understanding with the Cleveland Schools to supply their farming curriculum, where kids try to figure things out like how old the trees are and why compost heats up. They even put out a comic book that kids help to design and create. Whichever kid gives them the best idea is included in the comic book as a hero or shero. Rid-All is a demonstra-

> "For us, it's all about teaching kids to connect to the earth, and something that's ancient and tangible, not new and digital."
>
> —MARC WHITE

tion project; it's not viable commercially at this point. But that doesn't mean it isn't worthwhile. Just before I was leaving, Marc White, the site manager, said, "For us, it's all about teaching kids to connect to the earth, and something that's ancient and tangible, not new and digital."

The other program that really interested me is the Let's Move Salad Bars to Schools grant program. According to the Whole Kids Foundation, students who have access to a salad bar eat three times more fruits and vegetables! That's huge. Each salad bar cost $2,625, which includes all the component parts like chill pads and tongs. These bars last ten years. Maybe the USDA should give grants to school districts to do this? Wouldn't our Medicaid program be interested in doing this, too? In some schools 80 to 90 percent of the students are covered by Medicaid, the health program for the poorest in our society. If we consider what a really poor diet can do to a child's health, wouldn't having them eat more fruits and vegetables be a smart and economic move? Yes, it sounds a little wacky to suggest Medicaid pay for salad bars, but you know what? It would be more economical than what we're doing now. In my estimation, we need a garden in every school yard, a salad bar in every school lunch room, and a healthy kitchen in every schoolhouse.

■ ■ ■

WHAT YOU CAN DO

Parents have an amazing ability to teach their kids about good nutrition simply by being an informed resource at occasions that involve food. Meals eaten together are a great way to do this, so make it your goal to have a number of well-planned meals together each week. There are many resources to help with family meal planning online, as a simple Google search will show. I know a number of people who sit down on Friday night and go through recipes and pick out four of five for the upcoming week to save the stress of having to figure something out at the last minute. This leaves them with ample time to get the groceries and prep things over the weekend.

It's also helpful to get kids involved in grocery shopping and cooking. If they're allowed to make their own healthy eating and buying decisions, it will not only teach them about food, it will expand your eating perspectives as well.

Keep healthy food on hand and make it easy to grab. We cut up fruits and vegetables and keep them in a colander in the fridge, and the kids eat them because they are there and easily accessible. If you make unhealthy food harder to get, they are much less likely to eat it. This not only keeps them healthy, it trains their palates so they make good choices outside the home, too.

My wife, Andrea, is a fourth grade teacher. She has been concerned about the nutrition of the children she's been teaching for years. Some of the "meals" she's seen children bring to school have virtually no nutritional value. She started a small campaign to let her children eat in class, but only fruits and vegetables. Peer pressure can be a terrible thing, but it can also work to advantage. Now that kids have seen other kids with fruits and vegetables in class, they're asking their parents for them. Ask your children's teacher or principal to do the same as Andrea did.

If you aren't able to convince people of wholesale change within the school, it may be possible to create at least a onetime event, such as a classroom tasting party. Here you can bring in healthy foods that kids may not be familiar with and create an atmosphere of fun and exploration around eating well.

You can also download one or more of Jamie Oliver's toolkits to "start a Food Revolution at your school": www.jamieoliver.com/us/foundation/jamies-food-revolution/school-food. This will give you ideas on how to bring about change on your own.

The USDA has also been working to improve the food that our children eat in school. They've launched a Healthier U.S. School Challenge—at www.fns.usda.gov/hussc/healthierus-school-challenge-promo-materials—that rewards schools for offering healthier lunch options. You can check with your kid's school administration and encourage them to join and become a Team Nutrition School. The program offers training grants to school districts to assist them in promoting healthy eating.

Try playing simple games with your children like "How many vegetables can you name?" The website Sporcle offers a basic app for that at www.sporcle.com/games/Andy47/veggietables. There's also another one on the same site for naming all the different types of squash.

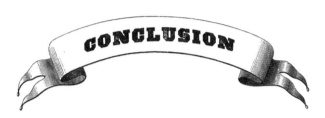

A NEW VISION
FOR AMERICA

Real food is not only about agriculture and nutrition. It's about a way of life that connects us back to the earth, to each other, to our communities, and to what really matters. It's about slowing down and really tasting life. It's about the joy of living.

> *What we plant in the soil of contemplation, we shall reap in the harvest of action.*
>
> —MEISTER ECKHART

On the surface, *The Real Food Revolution*—both the book and the revolution itself—appears to be about food policy. And in many ways, it is: what are the practical choices we are making, and are they sound? But it goes further and deeper than that. At its heart, this revolution is about the kind of life we want to have for ourselves and the kind of world we want to leave to our children. It is about a deeply satisfying kind of appreciation: for the amazing planet we have been given, the bounty and beauty it provides for us, and for the opportunity to be, for a very brief time, its stewards.

We experience these all-too-brief moments of appreciation when we're working in our garden; or sitting on the beach looking at the massive expanse of the ocean; or when we see a rainbow as the light from the sun breaks through a rainy day; or on those awesome nights when, far from the lights of the city, the stars are so bright we feel like we can reach up and grab one. These are peak experiences. *The Real Food Revolution* is extending the spirit of these momentary experiences of appreciation—when we have real reverence for life—into daily actions and behaviors. The revolution is working when those behaviors can become habits, for us and for our children, that will literally shift the landscape of America.

I wrote this book because of people I met who had a deep and abiding appreciation for quality of life, over and above efficiency and money. As Arianna Huffington has been saying in her Third Metric campaign and in her book *Thrive*, there is more to life than money and power. Without well-being, nothing is worth it. What do we really want out of this precious, rich life we have been given? In moments of deep reflection, what is most important to us? It seems to me that being deeply connected to the ones we love has to be at the top of most of our lists. Not too far behind is, probably, to just be connected. Not the technology type of connection that seems to plug our heads into some device, but the kind of connection you get in nature when you go for a hike or are planting flowers. The kind where your body relaxes and the wall your mind has built around you dissolves. As native peoples in so many cultures have long understood, we are part of the earth and the earth is part of us. We rest in our Mother's arms.

Our current food system has *dis*connected us from ourselves, our loved ones, and the earth. It has decreased our quality of life. It's apparent that we have a lot of knowledge today. We are the smartest people in history, or so it would seem. The problem is we have lost our wisdom. For millennia, the great religions drew wisdom from nature. The great spiritual teachers constantly used references to nature precisely because they were connected to it. Now that our society is disconnected from nature, not to mention each other, we are losing these common references that gave us our collective wisdom. While knowledge helps us survive, wisdom allows us to live. Let's start living again.

Having a seat belt on while eating a family dinner is not my idea of having quality time with the kids. Family dinners for generations kept the nuclear family connected. Let's bring them back. The family can be any kind of unit, just so long as people have community together, and young and old share common ground. The family dinner provides opportunities to bond, to laugh, to learn proper etiquette, to share, to chew your food with your mouth closed, to clean up after yourself, to lead the family in prayer. In the real food revolution and the slow food movement, the family dinner is a sacred ritual, and our food is the sacramental element.

The ritual of the family dinner is just one example of how we can slow down and reprioritize. And "family dinner" today doesn't need to be a throwback to the days of *Leave It to Beaver* or *Father Knows Best*. It can be a *Modern Family* dinner. It can mean potluck with friends. It could be a group of college students forming a cooking club and taking turns cooking for each other instead of eating fast food. It can be community gardeners sharing an outdoor feast together. It may be difficult for us to shift gears after building up so much momentum in the direction of finding the fastest and most convenient way to do things—the drive-through, takeout, ready-made life—but if everyone reading this just starts deciding to slow down where food is concerned, wouldn't that make it easier for the people in our circle and beyond? And maybe, just maybe, this can be the first step in slowing down our lives in other areas.

The real food revolution is about realizing we can help create a better, more enjoyable lifestyle for our families, our circle of friends, our colleagues at work, and ourselves. One that looks a lot like my grandparents' approach to living: fresh food, lots of cooking, happy hours, slow weekends with family and friends, and lots of laughter. It's like the old saying that nobody on their deathbed has ever wished they had spent more time at the office. It's a cliché, but it is absolutely true. And I think we could add that no one ever wished they ate faster and had more bad food, maybe the food that put them on their deathbed in the first place.

The real food revolution reconnects us to our land, as well. By growing our own food or knowing the farmer who has grown it, we connect back to the land. By connecting back we can start to embody the lessons that come with growing food. These same lessons also teach us how to behave in a civilized way. By being closer to nature we learn that anything worthwhile takes time. We cultivate fruits and vegetables for sure, but we also cultivate patience. And wouldn't our country benefit if we all had a little more patience? If we didn't expect things to change overnight? We sometimes fall into the trap of thinking that because a web page can pop up in one second, or because you can change the channel with a push of a button or heat up dinner in one minute, that everything should only take a minute. Staying connected to the land can keep front and center in our minds the universal truth that things take time.

If more and more Americans reconnected to each other and to the land, our public discourse might change for the better, as well. When it comes to planting gardens and crops, we learn just how true it is that we reap what we sow. And we can become aware of how this principle also operates in our personal lives. That awareness can help us govern our behavior and personal interactions accordingly, knowing that the seeds we plant today may come back to haunt us tomorrow. What a valuable lesson the earth teaches.

We also recognize that no matter how hard you work at cultivating a crop, it only feels truly rewarding if it is shared. And the same goes for cooking; not many people like to cook for just themselves. It is an act of generosity and fellowship. We can realize just the same that our time and talents in life only become deeply satisfying if they are shared. In the real food revolution, sharing and service to others is a guiding principle. In my experience, it is why farmers farm: to share with others.

A closer connection to the planet and our food system also gives us an appreciation for the different seasons of life. There is a time to plant, a time to water, and a time to reap the harvest. And while hoop houses and greenhouses can extend the life of the growing season, these timeless principles still remain. There will be good times and there will be bad. The older people I grew up with seemed to embody this understanding. I remember when my grandfather died, my grandmother, after 60-plus years of marriage, was terribly heartbroken. She died a few months later from a broken heart. But I remember her saying, even as she cried, "I'm not the first woman to lose her husband." She knew what season it was. She went through it with grace and dignity, even though she had a broken heart. And then she peacefully let go of her own life. Having a deep understanding of these laws of nature can help us along in life. The more we are in tune, the more we understand what season it is, the more graceful and dignified our lives will be.

While reconnecting to each other and the land is essential for us to transform the current food system, investments into research and technological development are critical to scaling up the new system to meet the challenge of feeding nine billion people by 2050. As *National Geographic* suggested in a video accompanying their "New Food Revolution" issue in May 2014, feeding the world is a complex problem with a lot of moving parts. One single solution will not do it, but too often that causes people to think that we should just turn it over to the smart people who will give us the next solution. But it's not so simple, as we've seen from all the unintended consequences that have come from genetically modifying our seeds. Under the current system, we serve the technology. In the real food revolution, technology needs to serve us. If we stay close to the land and embody the principle of staying connected to each other and to nature, we can make this work. Those values are the compass that keeps us going in the right direction.

Left to their own devices, the intellectual firepower in the food system today is going to figure out the next best genetically modified seed or how to get sugar, salt, and fat at the right levels to make us buy more quadruple-stuffed Oreo cookies. We need to challenge the next generation of scientists and engineers to help us design the techniques and equipment to ramp up a movement to deliver real food to all using sustainable methods. How we can develop reliable renewable energy to power up farms, fields, and gardens so we can keep their overhead low? Who is researching the new machine that can dig for different crops at the same time, so that farms with multiple crops can benefit from machinery as much as single-crop farms? How can we create incentives for more of our students to go into ag research directed at the new way of food production rather than preserving the status quo at all costs? How do we help poorer countries use technological advances to set up local and regional food systems? Let's figure out how to have advances in technology that help us create something much more inspiring than the latest nifty app: a new agriculture system that feeds us fresh, healthy food without damaging our environment.

As a former quarterback, I usually like to win. But as I have gotten older, my idea of how to achieve victory has changed. And one of my favorite books, Sun Tzu's *The Art of War*, has helped to reshape my worldview. It says, "Victory can be known. It cannot be made." I love that passage. I've come to understand that what it means is that victory is not necessarily something we fight and struggle for. It's something we find. Victory is a discovery. It's already right here. It's only a matter of finding it. In the real food revolution, we found it in the people we met from across this country who are changing the American food system, and we will continue to find it as we look out into our own communities. When it says victory is discovered, it is also suggesting that you don't yet know the precise solution to the problems you face today, but the solutions are there to be discovered if you point yourself in the right direction. We do not know *the* exact methodologies and solutions that will bring about a food system that isn't making us sick and damaging the very earth we walk on. But I feel strongly that we know the general direction. With the right intention and inspiration, we will see opportunities, solutions, and allies that we can't even imagine today. Let's heighten our awareness and open up to all the possibilities that will be emerging over the coming years.

One of my favorite commentators on *The Art of War,* James Gimian, says that we can "achieve our goals without resorting to aggression or engendering further conflict." That should be our mantra. There is enough aggression in the world today. We don't need to add to it. I've never believed that if we just got madder than the other side we would convince them to join us. If you want more love in the world, love. If you want more whole foods in the world, plant a garden. All the scream-ing in the world won't help. Let's vote with our dollars in the marketplace and at the ballot box. Let's use the Internet to push petitions and legislation that moves the cause forward. No drama, just action.

The real food revolution is grounded in the fact that we respect ourselves too much to just sit around and let a broken system serve us bad food indefinitely. We will focus, work, and organize until we get something better for our children. Not marginally better, but significantly better. A food system that is worthy of the deep affection and concern we have for the ones we love the most. We will slow down enough to see this. We will be of service to our fellow man. We will be thankful, we will be pa-tient, but all the while we will recognize that it is the time of the season for action.

I'd like to leave you with my vision for what I hope our food system will look like in the future.

It's a beautiful, sunny Saturday morning in Ohio, in late summer. The sky is clear and blue with an occasional fluffy white cloud above. My son Brady, who is ten years old, jumps into the backseat of our car, ready for our Saturday morn-ing ritual. "Bye, Mommy. I love you," he says as we put on our seat belts, pull out, and head up the road. After traveling about two miles, we pull into a rocky driveway that extends toward a big, old farm house. As dust kicks up all around us Brady reads the same sign as he does every week-end. "Farmers' Market," he says. "Hurry, Daddy!" As we drive past rows of hoop houses and green-houses sprinkled in this urban city block, Brady is waving at all his friends who are tending to the vegetables they grow on the 20 acres of land.

This is the Ed and Cathy O'Neill Organic Urban Farm, named after the actor who grew up in Youngstown and helped with an early donation to get things off the ground. It was purchased by the Youngstown Neighborhood Development Corporation about 15 years before. It started as a nonprofit that helped turn abandoned property in Youngstown, Ohio, into full-fledged urban gardens.

As we reach the old refurbished house on the farm, Brady jumps out of the car and runs into his sister Bella's arms. "Gooood morning, Brady!" she says as she kisses him all over the face. He beams and she tickles him. He giggles and runs over to scare the chickens.

Bella hugs me, and I ask her, "Whaddya have today?" She tells me that they have turnips and collard greens, and that the carrots look really good. "Nice, we'll take some of each," I say. "Why don't you put two bags together? Aunt April and Uncle Eric are coming over tonight for dinner." "No problem," she says.

Bella works at the farm when she is on summer break from college. She is studying to be an integrative health doctor. She has a deep passion for promoting healthy food and sustainable agriculture and understands that these are key to improving national health. So, she oversees the high school kids who work at this organic urban garden during the summer and gets a good tan, too.

She kisses Brady again and gives him a bag to carry. We're off to the next stop.

As we drive with the windows down, Brady starts eating a carrot freshly pulled from the ground, with the dirt he wiped off it still smeared on his face. A little dirt on his face won't kill him. He chomps away and tells me, "It's so sweet, Dad!" We're now surrounded by farmland. Brady starts to scream "Moooooo" out the window to the passing cows. They look back with deadpan stares. As we pull up to another farm, there's a huge red barn like the kind we used to have when I was growing up. While they disappeared for a while, the Ohio landscape is now littered with them again. "This farm is sustainable and we treat our animals humanely," Brady says out loud slowly as he reads the sign for McKinley Farm, a private, sustainable family farm that has a training program for young people who want to learn about humane and environmentally sound farming practices. "What does it mean, Brady, that the animals are treated humanely?" I ask. "The cows don't do drugs and the chickens don't sleep in poop," he says.

We park and walk over to see the cows. "Who is that?" I ask. Brady looks at me and smiles. I put my finger over my lip, making the *shhhh* sign. "Go sneak up on him," I whisper. A young kid about 20 years old is squatting by the side of a cow, attaching the pump that will get the milk out. Brady taps him on the shoulder and says,

"Can I get one cup from the front and one cup from the back?" "You little stinker!" his brother, Mason, says as he turns around and grabs a laughing Brady. He pretends he is going to toss him into a big pile of cow dung. "Easy!" I say. "If he slips, you're gonna be the one to wash his clothes."

"Come over here; I got something for you guys," Mason says. I love when he says that, because it always means something extra fresh is coming. "Look," he says, opening up the freezer, showing us a quart of fresh, homemade, organic peach ice cream. "We just picked the peaches and milked the cows yesterday." *Man, I love this kid,* I think. "How many can I buy?" I ask. "Two per customer," Mason says. "I caught holy hell when I let you buy eight last year." Okay. I have a weakness for ice cream. But this stuff is so creamy and fresh. No hormones. No antibiotics. From grass-fed cows. Delicious! He packs two in a bag with a couple of half-gallons of fresh milk. "The cheese isn't aged enough yet," he says. "But I have one more surprise. We just captured a ton of fresh honey."

"Nothing better than fresh honey," Brady says from across the barn while petting the cow, obviously repeating what he hears from me every time we get fresh honey. They look at each other and laugh. "Awesome. Thank you so much,"I say. We hug and head off.

Mason is getting his degree in sustainable agriculture and works here at McKinley Farm in the summer. He has become a real expert in all aspects of running a sustainable farm. The owner wants to make him part owner when he graduates. He and the owner have a patent pending on a new machine that can get milk from a cow using a pump that runs on the wind that comes from a windmill on top of the barn.

Next, we head to downtown Youngstown to make a quick stop at the Simeon Booker vertical farm (named after the Youngstown resident who was the most prominent journalist to chronicle the civil rights movement) to get lettuce, kale, and fresh tomatoes. I'm going to make my grandmother's pasta sauce tonight, and it's always best with fresh tomatoes. After pulling into a parking deck, we walk across a catwalk to the vertical farm. It is an old 18-story bank building that was converted to a giant greenhouse. It has an intricate watering system that recycles the water, uses solar power to energize the building, and supplies food to many of the downtown residents and restaurants.

The Youngstown Neighborhood Development Corporation (YNDC) built it with assistance from a U.S. Department of Agriculture grant. The technical expertise to do the project was supplied by the Ohio State University agriculture extension program. After a couple of years, the farm has become profitable and employs 15 people, 7 of whom are veterans. The bottom couple of floors are occupied by a Whole Foods Market. It's clean, the people are friendly, and they sell all the fresh fruits and vegetables they grow. Next door is Catullo Prime Meats, the

100-year-old local butcher shop that purchases all of their grass-fed cows and free-range chickens from local sustainable farms, including the one Mason works at. They process all of their meat humanely.

Within one block of the garden, there is a yoga studio, meditation hall, integrative health clinic, coffee shop, wine bar, Vernon's Italian restaurant, the OH WOW! children's museum, lots of loft housing, connection to a bike trail, and the downtown trolley system. The church across the street has even seen an increase in its congregation. An entire side of town that had been a food desert has become a gathering place of twenty- and thirtysomethings who live downtown, as well as empty nesters who have sold their homes in the suburbs and now rent.

After picking up some more vegetables and some chicken for soup, I walk Brady over to the children's museum to see what day his robotics camp starts. We then walk to Summer Gardens, a huge kitchen where they offer cooking lessons for up to ten people and wine tastings for many more. I want to pick up a schedule because I promised Andrea we'd go to a class on Northern Italian food. They use all the local food for their programs and they also partner with YNDC to train teachers who go out into community kitchens to teach people how to cook healthy, fresh, tasty food.

As we drive home, I notice in the rearview mirror that Brady has the ice cream out and it's all over his face. "What are you doing?" I say with faux sternness. "What?" he says. "It was melting. I had to do something! Haven't you always told me 'It's better to light a candle than curse the darkness'? Well?"

"So now you choose to listen to me? Pass it up here!"

Our Saturday ritual is my favorite time of the week.

Right now, I'm just using my imagination, but I feel optimistic that in ten years, much of what I've envisioned here *will be* a reality. And not just in Youngstown. With the determination and work of all the people profiled in this book—and you—we can make the dream of a healthier American food system come true. So join with me and the many others who are working toward this future. Together we can stand strong to create a healthier, happier America. For our generation and for hundreds more after us.

RESOURCES

A list of the available resources on the real food revolution that is taking place in this country, and the world over, could fill an entire book unto itself. I've chosen here to include a sampling of some of the many books, movies, podcasts, blogs, and web resources I've found valuable.

BOOKS

Food Crisis:

The Botany of Desire: A Plant's-Eye View of the World. Michael Pollan. Random House, 2001.

Cooked: A Natural History of Transformation. Michael Pollan. Penguin Group, 2014.

Eat, Drink, Vote: An Illustrated Guide to Food Politics. Marion Nestle. Rodale Books, 2013.

The End of Overeating: Taking Control of the Insatiable American Appetite. David Kessler. Rodale Books, 2010.

Fast Food Nation: The Dark Side of the All-American Meal. Eric Schlosser. Houghton Mifflin Harcourt, 2001.

Fat Chance: Beating the Odds Against Sugar, Processed Food, Obesity, and Disease. Robert Lustig. Hudson Street Press, 2013.

Food Fight: The Inside Story of the Food Industry, America's Obesity Crisis, and What We Can Do About It. Kelly Brownell and Katherine Horgen. McGraw-Hill, 2004.

Food Policy in the United States: An Introduction. Parke Wilde. Routledge, 2013.

Food Politics: How the Food Industry Influences Nutrition and Health. Marion Nestle. California Press, 2002 (revised 2013 with foreword by Michael Pollan).

Food Rules: An Eater's Manual. Michael Pollan. Penguin Group, 2014.

In Defense of Food: An Eater's Manifesto. Michael Pollan. Penguin Group, 2009.

The Industrial Diet: The Degradation of Food and the Struggle for Healthy Eating. Anthony Winson. UBC Press, 2013.

The Omnivore's Dilemma: A Natural History of Four Meals. Michael Pollan. Penguin Group, 2007.

Safe Food: The Politics of Food Safety. Marion Nestle. California Press, 2003 (revised 2010).

Secret Ingredients: The New Yorker *Book of Food and Drink.* David Remnick, ed. Modern Library Paperbacks, 2009.

What to Eat. Marion Nestle. Macmillan, 2006.

The World is Fat: The Fads, Trends, Policies, and Products that are Fattening the Human Race. Barry Popkin. Penguin Group, 2009.

Food System Flaws:

Empires of Food: Feast, Famine, and the Rise and Fall of Civilizations. Evan D. G. Fraser and Andrew Rimas. Simon & Schuster, 2010.

Food Justice (Food, Health, and the Environment). Robert Gottlieb and Anupama Joshi. MIT Press, 2013.

Foodopoly: The Battle Over the Future of Food and Farming in America. Wenonah Hauter. New Press, 2013.

The Meat Racket: The Secret Takeover of America's Food Business. Christopher Leonard. Simon & Schuster, 2014.

Pandora's Lunchbox: How Processed Food Took Over the American Meal. Melanie Warner. Scribner, 2014.

Salt Sugar Fat: How the Food Giants Hooked Us. Michael Moss. Random House, 2014.

Health:

The Anti-Inflammation Diet and Recipe Book: Protect Yourself and Your Family from Heart Disease, Arthritis, Diabetes, Allergies—and More. Jessica K. Black. Hunter House, 2006.

The Blood Sugar Solution 10-Day Detox Diet: Activate Your Body's Natural Ability to Burn Fat and Lose Weight Fast. Mark Hyman. Little, Brown and Company, 2014.

The Daniel Plan: 40 Days to a Healthier Life. Rick Warren, Daniel Amen, and Mark Hyman. HC Christian Publishing, 2013.

Eating Well for Optimum Health: The Essential Guide to Bringing Health and Pleasure Back to Eating. Andrew Weil. William Morrow, 2000.

Mindful Eating: A Guide to Rediscovering a Healthy and Joyful Relationship with Food. Jan Chozen Bays. Shambhala, 2009.

Savor: Mindful Eating, Mindful Life. Thich Nhat Hanh and Lilian Cheung. HarperOne, 2011.

True Food: Seasonal, Sustainable, Simple, Pure. Andrew Weil and Sam Fox, with Michael Stebner. Little, Brown and Company, 2014.

The UltraMind Solution: Fix Your Broken Brain by Healing Your Body First. Mark Hyman. Scribner, 2008.

Women's Bodies, Women's Wisdom: Creating Physical and Emotional Health and Healing. Christiane Northrup. Bantam, 2010.

Food Education

The Art of Eating: 50th Anniversary Edition. M. F. K. Fisher. Houghton Mifflin Harcourt, 2004.

The Cow in Patrick O'Shanahan's Kitchen. Diana Prichard (author), Heather Knopf (illustrator). Little Pickle Press, 2013.

Food Matters: A Guide to Conscious Eating. Mark Bittman. Simon & Schuster, 2009.

The Healthy Kitchen: Recipes for a Better Body, Life, and Spirit. Andrew Weil and Rosie Daley. Knopf, 2002.

Mindless Eating: Why We Eat More Than We Think. Brian Wansink. Bantam, 2013.

Slim By Design: Mindless Eating Solutions for Everyday Life. Brian Wansink. William Morrow, 2014.

Sweetness and Power: The Place of Sugar in Modern History. Sydney Mintz. Viking-Penguin, 1985.

What Makes the Crops Rejoice: An Introduction to Gardening. Robert Howard and Eric Skjei. Little, Brown and Company, 1986.

FILMS

Farmland. James Moll, dir. Allentown Productions, 2014.

Fat, Sick & Nearly Dead. Joe Cross, dir. Us & Us Media, Faster Production, 2010.

Fed Up. Stephanie Soechtig, dir. Atlas Films, 2014.

Food, Inc. Robert Kenner, dir. Magnolia Pictures, Participant Media, River Road Entertainment, 2008.

Forks Over Knives. Lee Fulkerson, dir. Monica Beach Media, 2011.

Fresh. Ana Sofia Joanes, dir. Ripple Effect Films, 2009.

The Future of Food. Deborah Koons Garcia, dir. Lily Films, 2004.

GMO OMG. Jeremy Seifert, dir. Compeller Pictures, Heartworn Pictures, Nature's Path, 2013.

Ground Operations: Battlefields to Farmfields. Dulanie M. Ellis, dir. and prod., 2013.

King Corn. Aaron Woolf, dir. ITVS, Mosaic Films, 2007.

Lunch Hour. James Costa, dir. Bird Street Productions, 2011.

Super Size Me. Morgan Spurlock, dir. The Con, Kathbur Pictures, Studio On Hudson, 2004.

PODCASTS

Freakonomics Radio. "You Eat What You Are" May 2012: freakonomics.com/2012/05/24/you-eat-what-you-are-part -1-a-new-freakonomics-radio-podcast

Ideas with Paul Kennedy. "Stuffed" December 2013: www .cbc.ca/ideas/episodes/2013/12/09/stuffed-part-1

The Splendid Table. Actor Wendell Pierce on opening a grocery store in a food desert in New Orleans: www.splendid table.org/story/actor-wendell-pierce-brings-grocery-stores -to-new-orleans

WEBSITES

Commentators:

Mark Bittman *The New York Times* blog: bittman.blogs .nytimes.com

Michael Pollan: michaelpollan.com

Food Policy:

Center for Food Safety: www.centerforfoodsafety.org

Civil Eats: civileats.com

CRS Report: What Is the Farm Bill? April 2014: www.fas .org/sgp/crs/misc/RS22131.pdf

Environmental Working Group—Farm Database: farm.ewg.org

Food and Environment Reporting Network: thefern.org

Food and Water Watch: www.foodandwaterwatch.org

Food Politics—Marion Nestle blog: www.foodpolitics.com

Rodale Institute: rodaleinstitute.org/our-work/research

U.S. Food Policy: A Public Interest Perspective (by Dr. Parke Wilde): usfoodpolicy.blogspot.com

USDA Center for Food Policy and Nutrition: www.cnpp .usda.gov

Diet and Health:

Dr. Andrew Weil: www.drweil.com

Dr. Christiane Northup: www.drnorthrup.com

Dr. Mark Hyman: drhyman.com

Harvard Nutrition Source: www.hsph.harvard.edu /nutritionsource

What We Eat in America, USDA Agricultural Research Service: www.ars.usda.gov/services/docs.htm?docid=13793

Yale Rudd Center for Food Policy & Obesity: www.yale ruddcenter.org

Food System Flaws:

Center for Ecoliteracy: www.ecoliteracy.org

Center for Science in the Public Interest: www.cspinet.org

Food Babe: foodbabe.com

Food Policy Action: foodpolicyaction.org/index.php

Food Tank: foodtank.com

The Lunch Tray: www.thelunchtray.com

National Sustainable Agriculture Coalition: sustainable agriculture.net

Urban Food/Local Farming:

Beginning Farmers: www.beginningfarmers.org

Brooklyn Urban Garden Charter School: www.bugs brooklyn.org

Cornucopia Institute: www.cornucopia.org

The Edible Schoolyard Project: edibleschoolyard.org

Growing Power: www.growingpower.org

The Intervale Center in Burlington, VT: www.intervale.org

Organic Consumers Association: www.organicconsumers.org

Riverpark Farm New York City: www.riverparkfarm.com /Riverparkfarm/farm.htm

Young Farmers Organization: www.youngfarmers.org

Food Education:

Choose My Plate: www.choosemyplate.gov

Eat Well: www.eatwellguide.org

Groceryships: www.groceryships.org

Jamie Oliver's Food Revolution: www.jamieoliver.com/us /foundation/jamies-food-revolution/home

The Kitchen Kid: www.kitchenkid.com

Let's Move: www.letsmove.gov

Slow Food USA: www.slowfoodusa.org

Whole Food Mommies: www.wholefoodmommies.com

BIBLIOGRAPHY

Much of the information, ideas, and insights in *The Real Food Revolution* comes from personal conversations with the people mentioned in the book and many others. Here are sources consulted for additional information and statistics.

Introduction

Size of Food Industry

- "Fortune 500 2014": fortune.com/fortune500/2014 (Figure for revenues for Fortune 500 companies in the food industry aggregate the revenues from the companies in the food services, food consumer products, beverages, and food production categories, and the grocery chains included in the food and drug store category. If chemical companies, such as Monsanto, were added in, the number would be higher.)

- Cantor, Stuart, ed. "Snack Trends 2013: Health and Indulgence Square Off." Food Processing: www.food processing.com/articles/2013/snack-trends

Obesity and Hunger:

- "Adult Obesity Facts." Centers of Disease Control and Prevention (March 28, 2014): www.cdc.gov/obesity /data/adult.html

- "Childhood Obesity Facts." Centers of Disease Control and Prevention (February 27, 2014): www.cdc .gov/healthyyouth/obesity/facts.htm

- "Hunger & Poverty Statistics." Feeding America: feedingamerica.org/hunger-in-america/hunger-facts /hunger-and-poverty-statistics.aspx#

PART I: THE PROBLEM

Chapter 1: Our Failing Health

Weight Gain: Nestle, Marion. *Eat, Drink, Vote: An Illustrated Guide to Food Politics.* (Rodale, 2013): 39.

Annual Sugar Intake: "Be a Sugar Detective." Yale Health: yalehealth.yale.edu/sugardetective

Increased Caloric Intake: Liebman, Bonnie. "The Changing American Diet." The Center for Science in the Public Interest, Nutrition Action Healthletter (September 2013): cspinet.org/new/pdf/changing_american_diet_13.pdf

Eating out vs. Eating at Home:

- "Food Expenditures." United States Department of Agriculture, Economic Research Service (April 15, 2014): www.ers.usda.gov/data-products/food -expenditures.aspx

Snacking:

- "Snacking Patterns of U.S. Adolescents." From What We Eat In America, NHANES 2005-2006, USDA Food Surveys Research Group, Dietary Data Brief No. 2 (September 2010): www.ars.usda.gov/SP2UserFiles /Place/12355000/pdf/DBrief/2_adolescents_snack ing_0506.pdf

- "Stuffed." *Ideas with Paul Kennedy.* Canadian Broadcasting Company, Toronto. December 9, 2013. Radio Podcast. (Note: Professor Popkin's statement of the number of bar codes for food products originally comes from this program, but he clarified in a June 2014 e-mail exchange that the starting figures were his estimates of the number of codes in the 1980s when no such data was collected.)

Nutrition and Mental Health:

- McCann, D., et al. "Food Additives and Hyperactive Behaviour in 3-Year-Old and 8/9-Year-Old Children in the Community: A Randomised, Double-Blinded, Placebo-Controlled Trial." *Lancet* 370, no. 9598 (November 3, 2007): 1560–67.

- Schab, D.W., et al. "Do Artificial Food Colors Promote Hyperactivity in Children with Hyperactive Syndromes? A Meta-Analysis of Double-Blind Placebo-Controlled Trials." *Journal of Developmental and Behavioral Pediatrics* 25, no. 6 (December 2004): 423–34.

- Weber, W., et al. "Complementary and Alternative Medical Therapies for Attention-Deficit/Hyperactivity Disorder and Autism." *Pediatric Clinics of North America* 54, no. 6 (December 2007): 983–1006.

Soda Consumption and Childhood Obesity:

- "Sugary Drinks and Obesity Fact Sheet." Harvard School of Public Health, The Nutrition Source: www .hsph.harvard.edu/nutritionsource/sugary-drinks -fact-sheet

- Bishop, Jennifer, et al. "ASPE Research Brief: Childhood Obesity." U.S. Department of Health and Human Services, Office of the Assistant Secretary for Planning and Evaluation (August 2005): aspe.hhs.gov/health/reports/child_obesity/index.cfm

Diet-Related Health Facts:

- Centers for Disease Control & Prevention: www.cdc.gov

- Choinière, Conrad, and Anu Mitra. "Consumer Diet-Disease Knowledge and Food Label Usage." *Consumers Interests Annual* 52 (2006): www.consumerinterests.org/assets/docs/CIA/CIA2006/choiniere-mitr_consumerdiet-diseaseknowledgeandfoodlabelusa.pdf

- "Leading Causes of Death." Centers for Disease Control and Prevention, National Center for Health Statistics (December 30, 2013): www.cdc.gov/nchs/fastats/leading-causes-of-death.htm

- Hyman, Mark. "Why ObamaCare Is Not Enough: It's the Health Care Costs, Stupid!" (February 21, 2013): drhyman.com/blog/2012/06/29/why-obamacare-is-not-enough-its-the-health-care-costs-stupid

- "The United States of Diabetes: Challenges and Opportunities in the Decade Ahead." United Health, Center for Health Reform & Modernization (November 2010): www.unitedhealthgroup.com/~/media/UHG/PDF/2010/UNH-Working-Paper-5.ashx

- "Diabetes Public Health Resource." Division of Diabetes Translation, National Center for Chronic Disease Prevention and Health Promotion (June 2014): www.cdc.gov/diabetes/?s_cid=cdc_homepage_topmenu_001

- "High Blood Pressure Facts." Centers for Disease Control and Prevention (July 7, 2014): www.cdc.gov/bloodpressure/facts.htm

- "Digestive Diseases Statistics for the United States." National Digestive Diseases Information Clearinghouse. *National Institutes of Health* 13–3873 (September 2013, updated online June 4, 2014): digestive .niddk.nih.gov/statistics/statistics.aspx

- "Irritable Bowel Syndrome." National Digestive Diseases Information Clearinghouse. *National Institutes of Health* 13–693 (September 2013, updated online June 25, 2014): digestive.niddk.nih.gov/ddiseases/pubs/ibs

- American College of Gastroenterology: gi.org

- Go, AS, et al. on behalf of the American Heart Association Statistics Committee and Stroke Statistics Subcommittee. "Heart Disease and Stroke Statistics—2013 Update: A Report from the American Heart Association." *Circulation* 127 (2013): e6–e245: www.heart.org /idc/groups/heart-public/@wcm/@sop/@smd /documents/downloadable/ucm_319587.pdf

- "Heart Disease Fact Sheet." Centers for Disease Control and Prevention: www.cdc.gov/dhdsp/data _statistics/fact_sheets/docs/fs_heart_disease.pdf

- "Heart Disease." National Center for Chronic Disease Prevention and Health Promotion, Division for Heart Disease and Stroke Prevention (February 5, 2014): www.cdc.gov/heartdisease/?s_cid=cdc_homepage _topmenu_001

- American Heart Association: www.heart.org

- Anand, Preetha, et al. "Cancer Is a Preventable Disease that Requires Major Lifestyle Changes." *Pharmaceutical Research* 25, no. 9 (September 2008): 2097–2116: www.ncbi.nlm.nih.gov/pmc/articles/PMC2515569

- "Cancer Prevention and Control." Division of Cancer Prevention and Control, National Center for Chronic Disease Prevention and Health Promotion (May 2014): www.cdc.gov/cancer/?s_cid=cdc_homepage _topmenu_001

- The British Association for Cancer Research: www .bacr.org.uk

- American Cancer Society: www.cancer.org

- International Agency for Research on Cancer: epic .iarc.fr/keyfindings.php

- Hyman, Mark. "Magnesium: The Most Powerful Relaxation Mineral Available." *Huffington Post* (January 15, 2010): www.huffingtonpost.com/dr-mark-hyman /magnesium-the-most-powerf_b_425499.html

- Hoy, Mary, and Joseph Goldman. "Potassium Intake of the U.S. Population What We Eat in America, NHANES 2009–2010." Food Surveys Research Group, Dietary Data Brief No. 10, (September 2012): www.ars.usda .gov/SP2UserFiles/Place/12355000/pdf/DBrief/10 _potassium_intake_0910.pdf

Chapter 2: Our Broken Environment

Increase in Food Production:

- Speedy, Andrew. "Global Production and Consumption of Animal Source Foods." *The Journal of Nutrition* 133, no. 11 (November 1, 2003): 4048S–4053S: jn.nutrition.org/content/133/11/4048S.full

- McGinnis, Laura. "Breeding and Genetic Change in the Holstein Genome." United States Department of Agriculture, Agricultural Research Service (2009): www.ars.usda.gov/is/AR/archive/oct09/genome1009 .htm

- "Putting Meat on the Table: Industrial Farm Animal Production in America." Pew Commission on Industrial Farm Animal Production: www.ncifap.org /_images/PCIFAPFin.pdf

- Gyles, Carlton. "Industrial Farm Animal Production." *Canadian Veterinary Journal* 51, no. 2 (February 2010): 125–128: www.ncbi.nlm.nih.gov/pmc/articles/PMC2808277

- Horowitz, Roger. *Putting Meat on the American Table: Taste, Technology, Transformation.* Johns Hopkins University Press, November 2005.

- Edgerton, Michael. "Increasing Crop Productivity to Meet Global Needs for Feed, Food, and Fuel." *Plant Physiology* 149, no. 1 (January 2009): 7–13: www.ncbi.nlm.nih.gov/pmc/articles/PMC2613695

- "Feed Grains Data: Yearbook Tables." United States Department of Agriculture, Economic Research Service: www.ers.usda.gov/datafiles/Feed_Grains_Yearbook_Tables/All_tables_in_one_file/fgyearbooktables full.pdf (Note: to convert tonnes/hectare to bushels /acre, go to www.agrimoney.com/calculator)

Fertilizer runoff: McAllister, C. H., P. H. Beatty, and A. G. Good. "Engineering Nitrogen Use Efficient Crop Plants: The Current Status." *Plant Biotechnology Journal* 10, no. 9 (2012): 1011–1025.

Hormones in Cattle and Sheep:

- Raloff, Janet. "Hormones: Here's the Beef." *Science News* 161, no. 1 (January 5, 2002): 10: www.phschool.com/science/science_news/articles/hormones_beef.html

- "FY08–FY10 Compliance and National Priority." United States Environmental Protection Agency (October 2007): epa.gov/oecaerth/resources/publications/data/planning/priorities/fy2008prioritycwa.pdf

- "An Urgent Call to Action: Report of the State-EPA Nutrient Innovations Task Group." State-EPA Innovations Task Group (August 2009): switchboard.nrdc.org/blogs/aalexander/Ex.%2012,%20U rgent%20Call%20(AR%201049-1218).pdf

- "Frequently Asked Questions about Veterinary Medicine." Food Standards Agency: http://food.gov.uk /business-industry/farmingfood/vetmeds/vetmedfaq

- Weil, Andrew. "Avoiding Hormones in Meat and Poultry?" Q & A Library: www.drweil.com/drw/u/id /QAA400066

Modern Farming—Factory Farms:

- Hribar, Carrie. "Understanding Concentrated Animal Feeding Operations and Their Impact on Communities." National Association of Local Board of Health (2010): www.cdc.gov/nceh/ehs/docs/understanding _cafos_nalboh.pdf

- "Factory Farm Nation: How America Turned Its Livestock Farms into Factories." Food & Water Watch (November 30, 2010): documents.foodandwaterwatch .org/doc/FactoryFarmNation-web.pdf

- Factory Farming: www.factory-farming.com

Industrialized Agriculture and the Environment:

- "Industrial Animal Agriculture: A Broken System. Fact Sheet." Pew Charitable Trusts (July 19, 2011): www .pewenvironment.org/uploadedFiles/PEG/Publica tions/Fact_Sheet/Pew-IndustrialAnimalAgriculture -BrokenSystem-July2011.pdf

- "Water Risk Management Research: Water Quality Research." United States Environmental Protection Agency: www.epa.gov/nrmrl/wswrd

- "National Water Quality Inventory Report to Congress." United States Environmental Protection Agency: water.epa.gov/lawsregs/guidance/cwa/305b

- "Overview of Greenhouse Gases." United States Environmental Protection Agency (April 17, 2014): epa .gov/climatechange/ghgemissions/gases/ch4.html

- "Risk Assessment Evaluation for Concentrated Animal Feeding Operations. United States Environmental Protection Agency (May 2004): nepis.epa.gov/Adobe/PDF/901V0100.pdf

- Michalak, Anna, et al. "Record-Setting Algal Bloom in Lake Erie Caused by Agricultural and Meteorological Trends Consistent with Expected Future Conditions." *Proceedings of the National Academy of Sciences of the United States of America* 110, no. 16 (April 16, 2013): 6448–6452: www.ncbi.nlm.nih.gov/pmc/articles/PMC3631662/#__ffn_sectitle

- Lawrence, Neal. "Danger on Tap: The Midwest's Water Is the Worst in the U.S.; Contaminant Pose Little-Known Risks to Your Family's Health." *Midwest Today* (Spring 1998): www.midtod.com/dangerontap.html

- "Water Quality." Grace Communications Foundation: www.sustainabletable.org/267/water-quality

- Fentress Swanson, Abbie. "What is Farm Runoff Doing to the Water? Scientists Wade in." *National Public Radio,* The Salt (July 5, 2013): www.npr.org/blogs/thesalt/2013/07/09/199095108/Whats-In-The-Water-Searching-Midwest-Streams-For-Crop-Runoff

Industrialized Agriculture and Pesticides:

- "Superweeds: How Biotech Crops Bolster the Pesticide Industry." Food & Water Watch (July 1, 2013): www.foodandwaterwatch.org/reports/superweeds

- Cassidy, Emily. "'Extreme levels' of Herbicide Roundup Found in Food." Environmental Working Group (April 18, 2014): www.ewg.org/agmag/2014/04/extreme-levels-herbicide-roundup-found-food

- Bøhn, T., M. Cuhra, T. Traavik, M. Sanden, J. Fagan, and R. Primicerio. "Compositional Differences in Soybeans on the Market: Glyphosate Accumulates in Roundup Ready GM Soybeans." *Food Chemistry* 153 (June 2014): 207–215.

- Krüger, Monika, Philipp Schledorn, Wieland Schrödl, Hans-Wolfgang Hoppe, and Awad A. Shehata. "Detection of Glyphosate Residues in Animals and Humans." *Journal of Environmental and Analytical Toxicology* 4, no. 2 (Jan 2014).

- McAllister, C. H., P. H. Beatty, and A. G. Good. "Engineering Nitrogen Use Efficient Crop Plants: The Current Status." *Plant Biotechnology Journal* 10, no. 9 (2012): 1011–1025.

Soil Erosion:

- "2007 National Resources Inventory." United States Department of Agriculture (2009): www.nrcs.usda .gov/Internet/FSE_DOCUMENTS/stelprdb1041379.pdf

- "Losing Ground." Environmental Working Group: www.ewg.org/losingground

Factory Farms and Threats to Biodiversity:

- "Honey Bees and Colony Collapse Disorder." United States Department of Agriculture: www.ars.usda.gov /News/docs.htm?docid=15572

- "FSA Pollinator Information." United States Department of Agriculture, Farm Service Agency (August 23, 2013): www.fsa.usda.gov/FSA/webapp?area=home&su bject=ecpa&topic=nra-pl

- Grzimek, B. *Grzimek's Animal Life Encyclopedia.* Van Nostrand Reinhold Co., New York (1975): www.ucmp .berkeley.edu/mammal/eutheria/chirolh.html

- "White-Nose Syndrome (WNS)." National Wildlife Health Center: www.nwhc.usgs.gov/disease_informa tion/white-nose_syndrome

- Hartzler, Robert G. "Reduction in Common Milkweed (*Asclepias syriaca) Occurrence in Iowa Cropland from 1999 to 2009." *Crop Protection* 29, no. 12 (December 2010): 1542–1544.

- Brower, Lincoln P., Orley R. Taylor, Ernest H. Williams, Daniel A. Slayback, Raul R. Zubieta, and M. Isabel Ramírez. "Decline of Monarch Butterflies Overwintering in Mexico: Is the Migratory Phenomenon at Risk?" *Insect Conservation and Diversity* 5, no. 2 (March 2012): 95–100.

Chapter 3: The Power of Government and Big Business

Farm Bill:

- "Agricultural Act of 2014: Highlights and Implications." United States Department of Agriculture, Economic Research Service (April 29, 20014): www.ers .usda.gov/agricultural-act-of-2014-highlights-and -implications.aspx

- "Newly Released Farm Subsidy Database Tracks Bloated Crop Insurance Subsidies." Environmental Working Group (May 22, 2013): www.ewg.org/policy -plate/2013/05/newly-released-farm-subsidy-data base-tracks-bloated-crop-insurance-subsidies

- EWG Farm Subsidies: farm.ewg.org/region .php?fips=00000

- Johnson, Renée, and Jim Monke. "What Is the Farm Bill?" Congressional Research Service (April 7, 2014): www.fas.org/sgp/crs/misc/RS22131.pdf

Ohio Diabetes Facts: "Ohio Diabetes 2010 Fact Sheet." *Ohio Department of Health* (March 4, 2011): www.odh.ohio.gov /~/media/ODH/ASSETS/Files/hprr/diabetes%20preven tion%20and%20control/ohiosdiabetesfactsheet.ashx

Lobbying and Political Pressure:

- Lipton, Eric. "Rival Industries Sweet-Talk the Public." *New York Times* (February 11, 2014): www.nytimes .com/2014/02/12/business/rival-industries-sweet-talk -the-public.html?_r=0

- "The Facts about High-Fructose Corn Syrup." Sweet-Surprise.com: sweetsurprise.com/western-sugar-litiga tion-case-history

- Center for Responsive Politics: www.opensecrets.org

- Boseley, S. "Political Context of the World Health Organization: Sugar Industry Threatens to Scupper the WHO." *International Journal of Health* 33, no. 4 (2003): 831–833: www.ncbi.nlm.nih.gov/pubmed/14758862

- Owens, Brian. "Storm Brewing over WHO Sugar Proposal." *Nature* (March 11, 2014): www.nature .com/news/storm-brewing-over-who-sugar-propo sal-1.14854

- Stiglitz, Joseph E. "The Insanity of Our Food Policy." *New York Times* (November 16, 2013): opinionator. blogs.nytimes.com/2013/11/16/the-insanity-of-our -food-policy

Chapter 4: Costs and Access

Organic vs. Non-organic Price Differences: www.mofga.org/Publi cations/MaineOrganicFarmerGardener/Fall2011/PriceDif ferences/tabid/1966/Default.aspx

Price Rise for Fruit and Vegetables and Drop for Sweeteners:

- Pollan, Michael. *In Defense of Food: An Eater's Manifesto* (New York: Penguin Group, 2009): 186.

- Nestle, Marion. "Does It Really Cost More to Buy Healthy Food?" Food Politics (August 5, 2011): www .foodpolitics.com/2011/08/does-it-really-cost-more -to-buy-healthy-food/

- Leonhardt, David. "Sodas a Tempting Tax Target." *The New York Times* (May 19, 2009): http://www.nytimes .com/2009/05/20/business/economy/20leonhardt .html

- Russo, Mike, and Dan Smith. "Apples to Twinkies 2013: Comparing Taxpayer Subsidies for Fresh Produce and Junk Food." USPIRG (July 2013): http://libflow .com/d/uodl7ahb/Apples_to_Twinkies_2013%3A _Comparing_Taxpayer_Subsidies_for_Fresh_Produce _and_Junk_Food

Declining Nutritional Value Due to Decline in Soil Quality:

- Mayer, Anne-Marie. "Historical Changes in the Mineral Content of Fruits and Vegetables." *British Food Journal* 99, no. 6 (1997): 207–211.

- Nestle, Marion. "Will Better Access to Healthier Foods Reduce Obesity?" Food Politics (April 30, 2012): www.foodpolitics.com/2012/04/will-better-access-to -healthier-foods-reduce-obesity

- Cummins, Denise. "How American Food Makes Us Fat and Sick." *Psychology Today* (June 14, 2013): www .psychologytoday.com/blog/good-thinking/201306 /how-american-food-makes-us-fat-and-sick

- Scheer, Roddy, and Doug Moss. "Dirt Poor: Have Fruits and Vegetables Become Less Nutritious?" *Scientific American* (April 27, 2011): www.scientificamerican .com/article/soil-depletion-and-nutrition-loss

- Davis, Donald. "Study Suggests Nutrient Decline in Garden Crops over Past 50 Years." The University of Texas at Austin (Dec 1, 2004): www.utexas.edu /news/2004/12/01/nr_chemistry

- Pollan, Michael. *In Defense of Food: An Eater's Manifesto* (New York: Penguin Group, 2009): 118–19.

Access to Healthy Food/Food Deserts:

- "Going Beyond Hunger: Food Insecurity in America." National Association for State Community Service Programs: nascsp.org/data/files/csbg_publications /issue_briefs/going-beyond-hunger-food-insecurity -in-america.pdf

- Block, D., and Kouba, J. "A Comparison of the Availability and Affordability of a Market Basket in Two Communities in the Chicago Area." *Public Health Nutrition 9*, no.7 (2006): 837–845.

- Bell, Judith, and Marion Standish, "Building Healthy Communities Through Equitable Food Access." *Community Development Investment Review 5*, no. 3 (2009): www.frbsf.org/community-development/files/bell_standish.pdf

- "Improve Access to Nutritious Food in Rural Areas." School of Government: www.sog.unc.edu/node/1940

- Treuhaft, Sarah, and Allison Karpyn, "The Grocery Gap: Who Has Access to Healthy Food and Why It Matters." The Food Trust (2010): thefoodtrust.org/uploads/media_items/grocerygap.original.pdf

- "Access to Affordable and Nutritious Food: Measuring and Understanding Food Deserts and Their Consequences." United States Department of Agriculture (June 2009): www.ers.usda.gov/media/242675/ap036_1_.pdf

- Jetter, K.M., and D.L. Cassady. "The Availability and Cost of Healthier Food Alternatives." *American Journal of Preventive Medicine 30*, no. 1 (January 2006): 38–44: www.ncbi.nlm.nih.gov/pubmed/16414422

- Morton, Lois Wright, and Troy Blanchard. "Starved for Access: Life in Rural America's Food Deserts." *Rural Realities 1*, no. 4 (2007): www.iatp.org/files/258_2_98043.pdf

Thrifty Food Plan: "USDA Food Plans: Cost of Food 1994–Present." U.S. Department of Agriculture: www.cnpp.usda.gov/usdafoodplanscostoffood.htm

Price Rise Differences: "Price Difference: Organic Versus Non-Organic; Store Versus Farmers' Market." *The Maine Organic Farmer & Gardener* (Fall 2011): www.mofga.org/Publications/MaineOrganicFarmerGardener/Fall2011/PriceDifferences/tabid/1966/Default.aspx

PART II: THE FIX

Chapter 5: A New View of Nutrition

Kris Carr:

- Stein, Lisa. "Living with Cancer: Kris Carr's Story" *Scientific American* (July 16, 2008): www.scientific american.com/article/living-with-cancer-kris-carr

- Carr, Kris: kriscarr.com

Gluten Intolerance: "Non-Celiac Gluten Sensitivity." Celiac Central: www.celiaccentral.org/non-celiac-gluten -sensitivity

Medical Education:

- Adams, K.M., M. Kohlmeier, and S.H. Zeisel. "Nutrition Education in U.S. Medical Schools: Latest Update of a National Survey." *Academic Medicine* 85, no. 9 (Sept 2010): 1537–42.

- UNC Gillings School of Global Public Health: sph.unc.edu/nutr/unc-nutrition

Nutrition:

- Choose My Plate, United States Department of Agriculture: choosemyplate.gov

- Weil, Andrew: drweil.com

Chapter 6: Policy Advocacy

Dan Barber:

- Blue Hill Farm: www.bluehillfarm.com/food/over view/team/dan-barber

- Cohen, June. "Q&A with Chef Dan Barber: Can Organic Farming Feed the World?" TED (March 17, 2010): blog.ted.com/2010/03 /17/qa_with_chef_da

- Barber, Dan. "What Farm-to-Table Got Wrong." *The New York Times* (May 17, 2014): www.nytimes. com/2014/05/18/opinion/sunday/what-farm-to -table-got-wrong.html

- NPR Staff. "'Third Plate' Reimagines Farm-to-Table Eating to Nourish the Land." (May 20, 2014): www. npr.org/blogs/thesalt/2014/05/20/313988991/third -plate-encourages-a-more-inclusive-eating-pattern

Hormones in Cattle and Sheep:

- Raloff, Janet. "Hormones: Here's the Beef." *Science News* (January 5, 2002): www.phschool.com/science /science_news/articles/hormones_beef.html

- "Are Hormones Used in Food Production?" Food Standards Agency (2006): www.food.gov.uk/business -industry/farmingfood/vetmeds/vetmedfaq /hormonesvetmed#.U3uhDNI7vJ8

- Weil, Andrew. "Avoiding Hormones in Meat and Poultry?" (October 31, 2006): www.drweil.com/drw/u/id /QAA400066

- Orlando, Edward, et al. "Endocrine-Disrupting Effects of Cattle Feedlot Effluent on an Aquatic Sentinel Species, the Fathead Minnow." *Environmental Health Perspectives* 112, no. 3 (March 2004): 353–358.

John Mackey: www.wholefoodsmarket.com/blog/john
-mackeys-blog

Seed Monopoly:

- "The GMO Seed Monopoly: Fewer Choices, Higher Prices." Food Democracy Now (October 4, 2013): www.fooddemocracynow.org/blog/2013/oct/4/the _gmo_seed_monopoly_fewer_choices_higher_prices

- Fernandez-Cornejo, Jorge, et al. "Genetically Engineered Crops in the United States." United States Department of Agriculture (February 2014): www.ers .usda.gov/publications/err-economic-research-report /err162.aspx#.Ux_m4_ldWCE

- "The Role of GE Seeds and Patent Systems." Center for Food Safety: www.centerforfoodsafety.org/issues/303 /seeds/the-role-of-ge-seeds-and-the-patent-system#

- Hilbeck, Angelika, et al. "Farmer's Choice of Seeds in Four EU Countries Under Different Levels of GM Crop Adoption." *Environmental Sciences Europe* 25 (2013): 12: www.enveurope.com/content/pdf/2190-4715-25 -12.pdf

- *Cargill*: www.forbes.com/companies/cargill

- Krebs, A.V. "Corporate Agribusiness: Monopolising Subsistence." www.converge.org.nz/pirm/corpag.htm

- Open Source Seed Initiative: www.opensourceseed initiative.org/about

- Benbrook, Charles. "The Magnitude and Impacts of the Biotech and Organic Seed Price Premium." *Organic Center Critical Issue Report* (December 2009): www .organic-center.org/reportfiles/SeedPricesReport.pdf

- Freese, Bill, and George Kimbrell. "Seed Giants vs. U.S. Farmers." Center for Food Safety and Save Our Seeds (2013): www.centerforfoodsafety.org/files/seed -giants_final_04424.pdf

Farm Subsidies:

- EWG Farm Subsidy Database: farm.ewg.org

- "Subtotal, Farming Subsidies in United States, 2012." EWG Farm Subsidies: farm.ewg.org/top_recips.php?fi ps=00000&progcode=totalfarm&yr=2012&regionna me=theUnitedStates

- "Price Loss Coverage Program: FAPRI U.S. and World Agricultural Outlook." Food and Agricultural Policy Research Institute: www.fapri.iastate.edu/outlook

- "Crop Insurance." United States Department of Agriculture, Economic Research Service (April 11, 2014): www.ers.usda.gov/agricultural-act-of-2014-high lights-and-implications/crop-insurance.aspx# .U7qQk_ldWSo

- Lavender, Mike. "Will Cotton Subsidies Ignite New Trade Dispute?" Environmental Working Group (January 24, 2014): www.ewg.org/agmag/2014/01/will -cotton-subsidies-ignite-new-trade-dispute

Antibiotics and Livestock:

- "Case Studies: How Unsafe Drugs Can Reach Patients." Pew Charitable Trusts (February 26, 2014): http://www.pewtrusts.org/en/research-and-analysis /issue-briefs/2014/02/26/case-studies-how-unsafe -drugs-can-reach-patients

- "Hogging It!: Estimates of Antimicrobial Abuse in Livestock (2001)." Union of Concerned Scientists (April 4, 2004): www.ucsusa.org/food_and_agricul ture/our-failing-food-system/industrial-agriculture /hogging-it-estimates-of.html

- "Questions and Answers: Summary Report on Antimicrobials Sold or Distributed for Use in Food-Producing Animals in 2011." U.S. Food and Drug Administration (February 5, 2013): www.fda.gov/ForIndustry/User Fees/AnimalDrugUserFeeActADUFA/ucm236149.htm

- "2009 Summary Report on Antimicrobials Sold or Distributed for Use in Food-Producing Animals." U.S. Food and Drug Administration: www.fda.gov/down loads/ForIndustry/UserFees/AnimalDrugUserFeeActA DUFA/UCM231851.pdf

- Keehn, Joel. "Improper Use of Antibiotics Kills Thousands and Harms Millions Every Year, CDC Says: Simple Steps in the Doctor's Office and the Supermarket Can Help Keep You Safe." *Consumer Reports* (September 16, 2013): www.consumerreports.org /cro/news/2013/09/antiibiotic-misuse-kills-thou sands-harms-millions/index.htm

- "10 Facts About Antibiotics, Resistance, and Food Animal Production." The Pew Charitable Trusts (May 2014): www.pewtrusts.org/~/media/Assets/2014/05 /HHIF10FactsFINAL.pdf

- "Antibiotic Resistance Threats in the United States, 2013." U.S. Department of Health and Human Services, Centers for Disease Control and Prevention (2013): www.cdc.gov/drugresistance/threat-report-2013/pdf /ar-threats-2013-508.pdf

Chapter 7: The Farm-to-Table Movement

GE Crops: Royte, Elizabeth. "The Post-GMO Economy: One Mainstream Farmer Is Returning to Conventional Seed—and He's Not Alone." *Modern Farmer* (December 6, 2013): modernfarmer.com/2013/12/post-gmo-economy

Vani Hari: Food Babe: foodbabe.com

Chapter 8: An Urban Food Revival

Alemany Farmers' Market: City and County of San Francisco: sfgsa.org/index.aspx?page=1058

New York City: "Farmers' Markets in New York City." State of New York Comptroller (August 2012): www.osc.state .ny.us/osdc/farmersmarkets_rpt6-2013.pdf

Detroit: The City of Detroit: www.detroitmi.gov

Will Allen/Growing Power:

- Growing Power, Inc.: www.growingpower.org

- Allen, Will. *The Good Food Revolution.* New York: Gotham, 2012.

Harry Rhodes/Growing Home: Boyce, Barry. "The Joy of Living Green." *Shambhala Sun* (November 2011): shambhalasun. com/index.php?option=com_content&task=view&id=37 75&Itemid=0.

Rid-All Green Partnership: www.greennghetto.org

Youngstown Neighborhood Development Corporation: www.yndc .org

Wendell Pierce: Rossetto Kasper, Lynne. "Actor Wendell Pierce Brings Grocery Stores to New Orleans." The Splendid Table: www.splendidtable.org/story/actor-wendell-pierce -brings-grocery-stores-to-new-orleans

Sterling Farms: sterlingfreshfoods.com

Rooftop Gardens:

- "Reducing Urban Heat Islands: Compendium of Strategies." Climate Protection Partnership Division, U.S. Environmental Protection Agency: www.epa.gov /heatisland/resources/pdf/GreenRoofsCompendium .pdf

- Liu, K., and B. Baskaran. "Thermal Performance of Green Roofs Through Field Evaluation." National Research Council of Canada. Report no. NRCC-46412 : archive.nrc-cnrc.gc.ca/obj/irc/doc/pubs/nrcc46412/nrcc46412.pdf

- Clark, C., Peter Adriaens, and F. Brian Talbot. "Green Roof Valuation: A Probabilistic Economic Analysis of Environmental Benefits." *Environmental Science and Technology* 42, no. 6 (February 9, 2008): 2155–2161.

Growth in Farmers' Markets: "Farmers Market Search." United States Department of Agriculture, Agricultural Marketing Service: search.ams.usda.gov/farmersmarkets

Little City Gardens: www.littlecitygardens.com

Chapter 9: Educating the Next Generation

Food Marketing to Children: "Food Marketing to Youth." Yale Rudd Center for Food Policy & Obesity: www.yaleruddcenter.org/what_we_do.aspx?id=4

Positive Messages:

- Jamie Oliver's Food Revolution: www.jamieoliver.com/us/foundation/jamies-food-revolution/home

- Hey Kids Let's Cook: heykidsletscook.com

- Whole Kids Foundation, Whole Foods: www.wholekidsfoundation.org

Salad in Schools:

- Kottke, T.E., N.P. Pronk, A. S. Katz, J.O. Tillema, and T. J. Flottemesch. "The Effect of Price Reduction on Salad Bar Purchases at a Corporate Cafeteria." *Preventing Chronic Disease* 10 (February 2013):120214

- "HealthierUS School Challenge." U.S. Department of Agriculture, Food and Nutrition Service: http://www .fns.usda.gov/hussc/healthierus-school-challenge

- "Salad Bar Nation." Whole Kids Foundation: www .wholekidsfoundation.org/get-involved/campaign /salad-bar-nation

Conclusion

Huffington, Arianna. *Thrive: The Third Metric to Redefining Success and Creating Well-Being, Wisdom, and Wonder.* New York: Harmony, March 2014.

National Geographic:

- Foley, John. "Feeding 9 Billion: A Five-Step Plan to Feed the World." *National Geographic*: www.national geographic.com/foodfeatures/feeding-9-billion

- "The Future of Food: How to Feed Our Growing Planet." *National Geographic:* food.nationalgeographic.com

Sun Tzu's Art of War:

- Tzu, Sun. *The Art of War: The Denma Translation.* Boston: Shambhala Publications, March 2001.

- Gimian, James, and Barry Boyce. *The Rules of Victory: How to Transform Chaos and Conflict—Strategies from the Art of War.* Boston: Shambhala Publications, March 2008.

- Gimian, James, and Barry Boyce. *The Simple Rules of Victory.* (Pamphlet) Halifax: SUCHNS, 2011.

ACKNOWLEDGMENTS

I would like to, first and foremost, thank the amazing team at Hay House publishing. They are a phenomenally professional organization that has a core mission of improving the quality of life for our citizens. Most especially, I want to thank the leaders at Hay House— Reid Tracy, president and CEO, and Patty Gift, director of acquisitions—for immediately encouraging me to make this book happen. From very early on they saw the positive impact it could have on our world and were relentless in their support.

Taking their lead, senior editor Laura Gray played a vital role in this process. Her strong interest in the topic area, steady hand, and constant enthusiasm and good cheer helped to make this book a reality. My dear friend and developmental editor, Barry Boyce, helped shape this project in a major way. I am always grateful for his unique ability to grasp the big-picture ideas that I sometimes have and help bring them down to the ground to be better understood and implemented. Our deep friendship and connection allowed this book to happen in an amazingly short period of time. Catherine Cho was a godsend as our chief researcher. Her thoroughness, dedication, and hard work were key to giving this book the scope that was needed to tie the entire revolution together. LeeAnn Heltzel's work on the graphics I will use in giving presentations on the book will help to accentuate key points and make more complicated ones clear. She is a real pro.

At key points, Matt Kaplan from my political team took time away from his day job on my campaign to pull things together for the book project. He's the kind of always-willing-to-pitch-in, go-to person any public servant would love to have on their team. And a special thanks to Pat Lowry, my current communications director and former high school teacher. He was the first person to really bring the importance of changing our food and food policy to my attention. And to Michael Julian, my agriculture legislative assistant in Washington, DC, for his great work over the years making sure we always focused on agricultural issues even though our congressional district has a small agriculture sector. His diligence helped me understand the complexities of our nation's food policy. I also need to thank my legislative and communications team for their honest critique of this work, including Ryan Keating, Michael Zetts, Anne Sokolov, Rick Leonard, and chief of staff Ron Grimes. In addition, a few people very knowledgeable on farm and food policy—including Scott Faber, of the Environmental Working Group; Mike Stranz of the National Farmers Union; Ferd Hoefner of the National Sustainable Agriculture Coalition; Jack Huerter, senior legislative assistant for the Senate Committee on Agriculture, Nutrition, and Forestry—provided critical insight in the final stages. And thanks to Jen Lynch, my former legislative director, for a very thorough review of the book from the perspective of the kind of farmers I want to support.

I owe a debt of gratitude to the scores of people I met with in the course of researching this book. They are in the vanguard of the real food revolution and it's their work I want to celebrate and give a boost to. Every one of them is mentioned in the book already. I just want to tip my hat to them here and wish them every success in their work.

Finally, to my best friend and wife, Andrea. Her constant support and encouragement were essential to this project, even when it meant my being away from home for extended periods of time. Her sense of humor and good cheer kept me going during some busy and tedious stretches that always come with writing a book while juggling other responsibilities. She was always interested and enthusiastic about this project. And as a thirty-something working mom who is concerned about public health and providing healthy food for our children, she was my first and most essential advisor on what this book should look like.

ABOUT THE AUTHOR

Tim Ryan was first elected to the U.S. House of Representatives in 2002, at the age of 29, and is currently serving in his sixth term representing Ohio's 13th congressional district. He is strongly committed to working for the economic and social well-being of his constituents in Northeast Ohio. He serves as a member of the powerful House Appropriations Committee, the committee that funds all federal departments and programs. He also serves as a member of the House Budget Committee and is cochairman of the Congressional Manufacturing Caucus; the House Caucus on Addiction, Treatment, and Recovery; and the Military Mental Health Caucus.

Ryan has been an outspoken advocate for changing the way our food system works and for promoting real food. He received the National Farmers Union Golden Triangle Award, the organization's highest legislative honor, in 2006, 2008, 2011, and 2012.

Before being elected to Congress, Ryan served in the Ohio State Senate. He currently lives in Northeast Ohio with his wife, Andrea, and their three children and two dogs.

We hope you enjoyed this Hay House book. If you'd like to receive our online catalog featuring additional information on Hay House books and products, or if you'd like to find out more about the Hay Foundation, please contact:

Hay House, Inc., P.O. Box 5100, Carlsbad, CA 92018-5100
(760) 431-7695 or (800) 654-5126
(760) 431-6948 (fax) or (800) 650-5115 (fax)
www.hayhouse.com® • www.hayfoundation.org

■ ■ ■

Published and distributed in Australia by:
Hay House Australia Pty. Ltd., 18/36 Ralph St., Alexandria NSW 2015
Phone: 612-9669-4299 • *Fax:* 612-9669-4144 • www.hayhouse.com.au

Published and distributed in the United Kingdom by:
Hay House UK, Ltd., Astley House, 33 Notting Hill Gate, London
W11 3JQ • *Phone:* 44-20-3675-2450 • *Fax:* 44-20-3675-2451
www.hayhouse.co.uk

Published and distributed in the Republic of South Africa by:
Hay House SA (Pty), Ltd., P.O. Box 990, Witkoppen 2068
Phone/Fax: 27-11-467-8904 • www.hayhouse.co.za

Published in India by: Hay House Publishers India, Muskaan
Complex, Plot No. 3, B-2, Vasant Kunj, New Delhi 110 070 • *Phone:*
91-11-4176-1620 • *Fax:* 91-11-4176-1630 • www.hayhouse.co.in

Distributed in Canada by: Raincoast Books,
2440 Viking Way, Richmond, B.C. V6V 1N2 • *Phone:*
1-800-663-5714 • *Fax:* 1-800-565-3770 • www.raincoast.com

■ ■ ■

Take Your Soul on a Vacation

Visit www.HealYourLife.com® to regroup, recharge, and reconnect with your own magnificence. Featuring blogs, mind-body-spirit news, and life-changing wisdom from Louise Hay and friends.

Visit www.HealYourLife.com today!